Complete Revision Notes for Medical Finals

Complete Revision Notes for Medical Finals

KINESH PATEL BA(Hons) MB BS
Senior House Officer
Department of Medicine
Hammersmith Hospital
London, UK

Hodder Arnold
A MEMBER OF THE HODDER HEADLINE GROUP

First published in Great Britain in 2006 by
Hodder Arnold, an imprint of Hodder Education
and a member of the Hodder Headline Group,
338 Euston Road, London NW1 3BH

http://www.hoddereducation.com

Distributed in the United States of America by
Oxford University Press Inc.,
198 Madison Avenue, New York, NY10016
Oxford is a registered trademark of Oxford University Press

Hodder Headline's policy is to use papers that are natural, renewable and recyclable products and made from wood grown in sustainable forests. The logging and manufacturing processes are expected to conform to the environmental regulations of the country of origin.

Whilst the advice and information in this book are believed to be true and accurate at the date of going to press, neither the author[s] nor the publisher can accept any legal responsibility or liability for any errors or omissions that may be made. In particular, (but without limiting the generality of the preceding disclaimer) every effort has been made to check drug dosages; however it is still possible that errors have been missed. Furthermore, dosage schedules are constantly being revised and new side-effects recognized. For these reasons the reader is strongly urged to consult the drug companies' printed instructions before administering any of the drugs recommended in this book.

British Library Cataloguing in Publication Data
A catalogue record for this book is available from the British Library

Library of Congress Cataloging-in-Publication Data
A catalog record for this book is available from the Library of Congress

ISBN-10 0 340 88943 8
ISBN-13 978 0 340 88943 5

1 2 3 4 5 6 7 8 9 10

Commissioning Editor: Georgina Bentliff
Project Editor: Jane Tod
Production Controller: Lindsay Smith
Cover Design: Nichola Smith
Cover Image: © Alfred Pasieka/Science Photo Library
Indexer: Laurence Errington

Typeset in 10 on 13pt Minion by Phoenix Photosetting, Chatham, Kent
Printed and bound in Spain

What do you think about this book? Or any other Hodder Arnold title?
Please visit our website: www.hoddereducation.com

Contents

To my parents

Contributors

Simon R J Bott FRCS
Specialist Registrar in Urology, South Thames Region, London, UK

Alex Charkin BSc(Hons) MB BS MRCS DOHNS
Senior House Officer in Ear, Nose and Throat, St George's Hospital, London, UK

Ben Eddy MRCS
Specialist Registrar in Urology, South Thames Region, London, UK

Jagdeep Singh Gandhi BSc(Hons) MB ChB MRCS MRCOphth
Specialist Registrar in Ophthalmology, The Royal Eye Hospital, Manchester, UK

Gareth G Jones BSc(Hons) MB BS
Senior House Officer in Orthopaedics, Kingston Hospital, London, UK

Alexandra Kent MB ChB MRCP
Specialist Registrar in Gastroenterology, St Mary's Hospital, London, UK

Julian Leong MA(Oxon) MB BS MRCS(Eng)
Clinical Research Fellow, Imperial College London, UK

Kinesh Patel BA(Hons) MB BS
Senior House Officer, Department of Medicine, Hammersmith Hospital, London, UK

Natasha H Patel BSc(Hons) MB BS MRCP
Specialist Registrar in Diabetes and Endocrinology, North West Thames Rotation, London, UK

Simon Phillips BSc(Hons) MB BS MRCS
Specialist Registrar in Surgery, Dorset County Hospital, Dorchester, Dorset, UK

Kirstin Satherley BSc(Hons) MB BS MRCP
Specialist Registrar in Clinical Oncology, The Royal Marsden Hospital, London, UK

Preface

Finals tend to be a stressful time for medical students, as the requirement to relearn the large volumes of knowledge accumulated over five or six years is demanding, both physically and emotionally. Often the most difficult part is deciding exactly what level of detail is expected by examiners: the constant fear of not knowing enough inevitably leads students to try to learn too much from complicated texts, and consequently the key points that examiners actually seek are often forgotten.

This book is useful, as it uniquely contains the entire undergraduate curriculum examined at finals, from medicine to surgery and ENT to oncology. The salient points needed to pass are featured in an easy to read (and remember!) bulleted format.

As most examinations are now multiple choice question-based, these bullets provide the essential nuggets of information that are often difficult and time-consuming to extract from a conventional textbook. Particular thought has been given to include facts that are repeatedly tested in finals, though explanations have been kept deliberately brief to act more as an aide-mémoire than to provide comprehensive descriptions of diseases.

The content is deliberately broad, but without the unnecessary extensive verbosity that can create real confusion and anxiety in the days running up to exams. The information contained within this book should be sufficient to pass written finals.

I wish you every success in your studies.

Kinesh Patel

Acknowledgements

I would like to thank all the staff at Hodder for their help and encouragement, especially Georgina Bentliff without whose faith this project would never have been possible.

List of icons

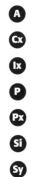

A Aetiology/incidence

Cx Complications

Ix Investigations

P Pathology

Px Prognosis

Si Signs

Sy Symptoms

S Signs and symptoms

Rx Treatment

Abbreviations

AAA	abdominal aortic aneurysm
AAFB	acid- and alcohol-fast bacilli
Ab	antibody
ABC	airway, breathing, circulation
ABG	arterial blood gases
ABPI	ankle brachial pressure index
ACA	anticentromere antibody
ACE	angiotensin-converting enzyme
ACS	acute coronary syndrome
ACTH	adrenocorticotrophic hormone
AD	Alzheimer's disease
ADH	antidiuretic hormone
AE	acute endocarditis
AF	atrial fibrillation
AFB	acid-fast bacilli
Ag	antigen
AGN	acute glomerulonephritis
AIDS	acquired immune deficiency syndrome
AIH	autoimmune hepatitis
AIHA	autoimmune haemolytic anaemia
AITP	autoimmune thrombocytopenic purpura
ALP	alkaline phosphatase
ALS	amyotrophic lateral sclerosis
ALT	alanine transaminase
AMA	antimitochondrial antibody
AML	acute myelogenous leukaemia
ANA	antinuclear antibodies
ANCA	antineutrophil cytoplasmic antibodies
AP	anteroposterior
APKD	adult polycystic kidney disease
APTT	activated partial thromboplastin time
APUD	amine precursor uptake and decarboxylation
ARDS	acute respiratory distress syndrome
ARF	acute renal failure

5-ASA	5-aminosalicylic acid
ASD	atrial septal defect
ASIS	anterior superior iliac spine
ASO	antistreptolysin O
AST	aspartate transaminase
ATLS	advanced trauma life support
ATN	acute tubular necrosis
AV	atrioventricular (node)
AVB	atrioventricular block
AXR	abdominal X-ray
BaFT	barium follow-through
BAL	broncho-alveolar lavage
BCC	basal cell carcinoma
BE	base excess
BMI	body mass index
BP	blood pressure
BPH	benign prostatic hyperplasia
BT	breath test
CBD	common bile duct
CCF	congestive cardiac failure
CCP	cyclic citrullinated peptide
CFA	cryptogenic fibrosing alveolitis
CFU	colony-forming units
CJD	Creutzfeldt–Jakob disease
CK	creatine kinase
CML	chronic myeloid leukaemia
CMV	cytomegalovirus
CNS	central nervous system
COMT	catechol O-methyltransferase
COPD	chronic obstructive pulmonary disease
CPN	common peroneal nerve
CrCl	creatinine clearance
CRF	chronic renal failure
CRP	C-reactive protein
CSF	cerebrospinal fluid
CT	computed tomography
CTPA	CT pulmonary angiography
CTR	cardiothoracic ratio
CVA	cerebrovascular accident
CVP	central venous pressure
CVS	cardiovascular system
CXR	chest X-ray
DCIS	ductal carcinoma *in situ*
DDH	developmental dysplasia of the hip
DEXA	dual-energy X-ray absorptiometry
DI	diabetes insipidus
DIC	disseminated intravascular coagulation

DIP	distal interphalangeal joint
DM	diabetes mellitus
DMARD	disease-modifying antirheumatic drugs
DVT	deep vein thrombosis
EAA	extrinsic allergic alveolitis
EBV	Epstein–Barr virus
ECF	extracellular fluid
ECG	electrocardiogram
EEG	electroencephalogram
EMG	electromyogram
ERCP	endoscopic retrograde cholangiopancreatography
ESR	erythrocyte sedimentation rate
ESRF	end-stage renal failure
ESWL	extracorporeal shockwave lithotripsy
EUA	examination under anaesthesia
FAP	familial adenomatous polyposis coli syndrome
FBC	full blood count
FDP	fibrin degradation products
FEV_1	forced expiratory volume in 1 s
FFP	fresh-frozen plasma
FHH	familial hypocalciuric hypercalcaemia
FNA	fine needle aspiration
FSGS	focal segmental glomerulosclerosis
FSH	follicle-stimulating hormone
5-FU	5-fluorouracil
FVC	forced vital capacity
GA	general anaesthetic
GBM	glomerular basement membrane
GCS	Glasgow Coma Score
G-CSF	granulocyte colony-stimulating factor
GFR	glomerular filtration rate
GGT	gamma glutamyl transferase
GH	growth hormone
GI	gastrointestinal
GM-CSF	granulocyte monocyte colony-stimulating factor
GN	glomerulonephritis
GnRH	gonadotrophin-releasing hormone
GOJ	gastro-oesophageal junction
GORD	gastro-oesophageal reflux disease
GP	general practitioner
G6PD	glucose-6-phosphate dehydrogenase
GTN	glyceryl trinitrate
HAART	highly active antiretroviral treatment
HAV	hepatitis A virus
Hb	haemoglobin
HbA_{1c}	haemoglobin A_{1c}
HBV	hepatitis B virus

HBcAb	hepatitis B core antibody
HBcAg	hepatitis B core antigen
HBeAb	hepatitis B e antibody
HBeAg	hepatitis B e antigen
HBsAb	hepatitis B surface antibody
HBsAg	hepatitis B surface antigen
HCC	hepatocellular carcinoma
HCG	human chorionic gonadotrophin
HCV	hepatitis C virus
HD	Huntingdon's disease
HDV	hepatitis D virus
HEV	hepatitis E virus
HF	heart failure
HHC	hereditary haemochromatosis
5-HIAA	5-hydroxyindoleacetic acid
HIV	human immunodeficiency virus
HLA	human leucocyte antigen
HMSN	hereditary motor and sensory neuropathy
HNPCC	hereditary non-polyposis colon cancer
HOCM	hypertrophic obstructive cardiomyopathy
HONK	hyperosmolar non-ketotic coma
HPV	human papillomavirus
HR	heart rate
HRT	hormone replacement therapy
HRCT	high-resolution CT
HSV	herpes simplex virus
5-HT	5-hydroxytryptamine
HTLV-1	human T-cell lymphotropic virus type 1
HUS	haemolytic uraemic syndrome
HZV	herpes zoster virus
IBD	inflammatory bowel disease
ICF	intracellular fluid
ICP	intracranial pressure
IF	intrinsic factor
IFG	impaired fasting glycaemia
IGF	insulin-like growth factor
IgG	immunoglobulin G
IgM	immunoglobulin M
IGT	impaired glucose tolerance
IHD	ischaemic heart disease
i.m.	intramuscular
INR	international normalized ratio
IPF	idiopathic pulmonary fibrosis
ITP	idiopathic thrombocytopenic purpura
ITU	intensive therapy unit
i.v.	intravenous
IVC	inferior vena cava

IVDU	intravenous drug use
IVU	intravenous urogram
JVP	jugular venous pressure
KUB	kidneys, ureter and bladder
LA	left atrium
LA	local anaesthetic
LDH	lactate dehydrogenase
LDL	low-density lipoprotein
LFT	liver function tests
LH	luteinizing hormone
LIF	left iliac fossa
LKM	liver, kidney, microsomal antibody
LMWH	low molecular weight heparin
LOS	lower oesophageal sphincter
LP	lumbar puncture
LUQ	left upper quadrant
LV	left ventricle/ventricular
MAC	*Mycobacterium avium* complex
MC&S	microscopy, culture and sensitivity
MCV	mean corpuscular volume
MDR-TB	multi-drug-resistant TB
MDT	multidisciplinary team
MEN	multiple endocrine neoplasia
MI	myocardial infarction
MIBG	metaiodobenzylguanidine
MLF	medial longitudinal fasciculus
MMR	measles, mumps and rubella
MR	mitral regurgitation
MRA	magnetic resonance angiography
MRCP	MR cholangiopancreatography
MRI	magnetic resonance imaging
MRSA	methicillin-resistant *Staphylococcus aureus*
MS	multiple sclerosis
MSU	mid-stream urine
MTP	metatarsophalangeal joint
NASH	non-alcoholic steatohepatitis
NBM	nil by mouth
NCS	nerve conduction studies
NGT	nasogastric tube
NHL	non-Hodgkin's lymphoma
NIPPV	non-invasive positive pressure ventilation
NNRTI	non-nucleoside reverse transcriptase inhibitors
NNT	number needed to treat
NPV	negative predictive value
NRTI	nucleoside reverse transcriptase inhibitor
NSAID	non-steroidal anti-inflammatory drug
NSTEMI	non-ST-elevation myocardial infarction

OA	osteoarthritis
OCP	oral contraceptive pill
OGD	oesophagogastroduodenoscopy
OGTT	oral glucose tolerance test
OI	opportunistic infection
ORIF	open reduction and internal fixation
OT	occupational therapy
PBC	primary biliary cirrhosis
P_{CO_2}	partial pressure of carbon dioxide
PCP	*Pneumocystis carinii* pneumonia
PCR	polymerase chain reaction
PD	Parkinson's disease
PE	pulmonary embolism
PEFR	peak expiratory flow rate
PET	positron emission tomography
PH	pulmonary hypertension
PICA	posterior inferior cerebellar artery
P_{O_2}	partial pressure of oxygen
POP	plaster of Paris
PPH	primary pulmonary hypertension
PPI	proton pump inhibitor
PPV	positive predictive value
PR	per rectum
prn	pro re nata
PRV	polycythaemia rubra vera
PSA	prostate-specific antigen
PSC	primary sclerosing cholangitis
PT	prothrombin time
PTCA	percutaneous transluminal coronary angioplasty
PTH	parathyroid hormone
PTHrP	PTH-related peptide
PUJ	pelvic–ureteric junction
PUVA	psoralen plus ultraviolet A
RA	right atrium
RA	rheumatoid arthritis
RBBB	right bundle branch block
RBC	red blood cell
RCC	renal cell carcinoma
RhF	rheumatoid factor
RIF	right iliac fossa
RR	respiration rate
RT	radiotherapy
RUQ	right upper quadrant
RV	right ventricle
SAH	subarachnoid haemorrhage
SBE	subacute bacterial endocarditis
SCC	squamous cell carcinoma

SCLC	small cell lung carcinoma
SeHCAT	selenium-75-homocholic acid taurine
SIADH	syndrome of inappropriate antidiuretic hormone
SLE	systemic lupus erythematosus
SOB	shortness of breath
SPECT	single photon emission computed tomography
SSRI	selective serotonin reuptake inhibitor
STEMI	ST-elevation myocardial infarction
SVC	superior vena cava
T_3	tri-iodothyronine
T_4	thyroxine
TB	tuberculosis
TCC	transitional cell carcinoma
TED	thromboembolic deterrent
TFT	thyroid function tests
TIA	transient ischaemic attack
TIBC	total iron binding capacity
TIPS	transjugular intrahepatic portosystemic shunt
TJ	transjugular
TNF-α	tissue necrosis factor-α
TNM	tumour, node, metastasis
TPHA	*Treponema pallidum* haemagglutination assay
TPN	total parenteral nutrition
TSH	thyroid-stimulating hormone
TT	thrombin time
tTG	tissue transglutaminase
TURP	trans-urethral resection of the prostate
UDCA	ursodeoxycholic acid
U&E	urea and electrolytes
USS	ultrasound scan
URTI	upper respiratory tract infection
UTI	urinary tract infection
UVB	ultraviolet B
VATS	video-assisted thoracic surgery
VDRL	venereal diseases research laboratory
VF	ventricular fibrillation
VIP	vasoactive intestinal peptide
$\dot{V}/\dot{Q}$	ventilation–perfusion
VRE	vancomycin-resistant enterococcus
VSD	ventricular septal defect
VT	ventricular tachycardia
VUJ	vesico–ureteric junction
vWF	von Willebrand factor
WBC	white blood cell
WCC	white cell count
WLE	wide local excision
WPW	Wolff–Parkinson–White syndrome

CHAPTER 1

Medicine

Alexandra Kent and Natasha Patel

CARDIOLOGY

CARDIAC INVESTIGATIONS

- **ECG (electrocardiography):** records cardiac electrical activity
- **Echocardiography (echo):** ultrasound imaging of the heart which gives a good impression of cardiac chambers, valvular heart disease, the pericardium, great vessels and masses; *transthoracic echo* is quick and easy to perform, but *trans-oesophageal echo* gives more detailed images, especially of the posterior structures
- **Doppler echocardiography:** Doppler studies measure the velocity and direction of red blood flow, and are useful for assessing flow across valves, through the great vessels and through cardiac chambers
- **Stress echocardiography:** echo is done at baseline, then immediately after exercise or dobutamine infusion (which increases myocardial oxygen demand); systolic function and regional wall motion abnormalities are recorded to assess for myocardial ischaemia
- **Nuclear imaging:** thallium or technetium-labelled compounds can be used to assess ventricular function and myocardial ischaemia; at rest and during stress; **SPECT (single photon emission computed tomography)** and **PET (positron emission tomography)** are being increasingly used
- **MRI (magnetic resonance imaging)/CT (computed tomography):** used to define anatomy; useful in congenital heart disease, tumours, pericardial disease; **MRA (MR angiography)** can be used to assess the aorta, large vessels and myocardial perfusion
- **Cardiac catheterization:** involves passage of a catheter from a peripheral artery into the heart for pressure measurements or injection of a contrast agent; angiography can assess the left ventricle, coronary arteries and aorta; allows for balloon angioplasty or stent insertion

HEART FAILURE (HF)

(P) Occurs when the heart is unable to pump blood at a rate required by metabolizing tissues

(A) Ischaemic, valvular, hypertensive or congenital heart disease, cardiomyopathy, myocarditis, endocarditis, pulmonary embolism (PE)
Precipitating factors: myocardial infarction, infection, arrhythmia, anaemia, thyrotoxicosis, electrolyte disturbance, PE, pregnancy

(S) *Left-sided heart failure (HF)*: dyspnoea, orthopnoea, paroxysmal nocturnal dyspnoea, fatigue, lung crepitations, pleural effusions, cyanosis
Right-sided HF: peripheral oedema, abdominal distension/ascites, tender pulsatile hepatomegaly, ↑ jugular venous pressure (JVP), hepatojugular reflux
Severe HF: reduced pulse pressure, hypotension, cool peripheries, 3rd ± 4th heart sounds, gallop rhythm

(Ix) Full blood count (FBC), urea and electrolytes (U&E), liver function tests (LFT), lipid profile, thyroid function tests (TFT), glucose, cardiac enzymes, ECG, chest X-ray (CXR), echo with colour Doppler studies

(Rx) Treat any risk factor (cholesterol reduction, glycaemic control, weight loss, smoking cessation etc.); remove any precipitant
Diuretics, angiotensin-converting enzyme (ACE) inhibitors or angiotensin receptor blockers, β-blockers, digoxin, glyceryl trinitrate (GTN) infusion

ISCHAEMIC HEART DISEASE

(P) Ischaemia occurs whenever there is an imbalance between oxygen delivery and oxygen demand; the commonest lesion is the atherosclerotic plaque
Ischaemia can also occur when coronary blood flow is limited – coronary spasm, emboli, aortic stenosis with left ventricular (LV) hypertrophy
It can be precipitated by severe anaemia (due to ↓ oxygen-carrying capacity of the blood)

(A) Obesity, smoking, insulin resistance/Type 2 diabetes mellitus, high-fat diet, hypertension, high cholesterol/low-density lipoprotein (LDL)
Ischaemic heart disease (IHD) is the most common cause of death in the developed world

ACUTE CORONARY SYNDROME (ACS)

This encompasses **angina, unstable angina** and **non-ST-elevation myocardial infarction (NSTEMI)**

(S) Central crushing chest pain, ± radiation to neck and left arm, sweating, dyspnoea, pallor

(Ix) FBC, U&E, glucose, lipids, cardiac enzymes, CXR, ECG (T wave inversion, ST depression), exercise testing, stress echo/nuclear imaging if patient unable to exercise, ± coronary angiography

(Rx) *Acute presentation*: oxygen, GTN spray, aspirin, clopidogrel, low molecular weight heparin (LMWH), ± GTN infusion, glycoprotein IIb/IIIa inhibitors (e.g. tirofiban)
Long term treatment: nitrates, β-blockers, calcium channel antagonists, aspirin, clopidogrel (for up to 1 year following non-ST elevation myocardial infarction [MI]), nicorandil; coronary revascularization

---

Box 1.1 GRADING OF ANGINA

I	angina on strenuous or prolonged exertion
II	slight limitation of ordinary activity; angina on moderate activity
III	marked limitation of ordinary activity; angina on mild activity
IV	unable to carry out activities without angina; may occur at rest

Source: Campeau L. Grading of angina pectoris [letter]. *Circulation* 1976;54:522–3 (reproduced with kind permission by the Canadian Cardiovascular Society)

ST-ELEVATION MYOCARDIAL INFARCTION (STEMI)

(P) Usually occurs due to atherosclerotic plaque rupture, leading to thrombosis formation, and coronary artery occlusion

(Sy) Similar to that of ACS, but more severe

(Ix) As for ACS; ECG will show ST segment elevation and Q waves evolve
Echo will indicate myocardial damage with abnormal wall motion

(Rx) *Acute presentation:* oxygen, GTN spray, aspirin, clopidogrel, primary percutaneous transluminal coronary angioplasty (PTCA), fibrinolysis (if PTCA not available)
Long term management: β-blockers, ACE inhibitors, aspirin, statins

(Cx) Heart failure, cardiogenic shock, arrhythmias, pericarditis, ventricular septal rupture, recurrent pain, LV aneurysm

HYPERTENSION

(P) Defined as blood pressure >140/90 mmHg

Box 1.2 CLASSIFICATION OF HYPERTENSION

- *Essential hypertension*: arterial hypertension with no specific cause; >90 per cent of cases
- *Secondary hypertension*: due to conditions including:
  - endocrine disorders
      Cushing's syndrome
      phaeochromocytoma
      acromegaly
      Conn's syndrome
      thyrotoxicosis
  - renal disease
  - acute porphyria
  - coarctation of the aorta
  - iatrogenic
      ciclosporin
      contraceptives
      steroids

(A) Obesity, salt intake, alcohol, diabetes mellitus, genetic inheritance

(Sy) Headaches, dizziness, blurred vision, epistaxis, angina, syncope, signs of heart failure ± symptoms related to underlying causes

(Si) LV heave, 4th heart sound ± 3rd heart sound, hypertensive retinopathy, carotid/renal bruits

Ix FBC, U&E, fasting glucose and lipid profile, haemoglobin A_{1c} (HbA$_{1c}$), urine for sugar/protein/blood/creatinine clearance, ECG (LV hypertrophy ± strain), CXR
Other investigations would be to rule out secondary causes e.g. calcium, TFT, cortisol, dexamethasone suppression test (Cushing's), 24-h urine for hydroxyindoleacetic acid (HIAA) (carcinoid)/catecholamines (phaeochromocytoma), aldosterone:renin ratio (Conn's syndrome), renal Doppler flow studies, renal MRA (renal artery stenosis)

Rx *Lifestyle*: weight loss, salt restriction, stop smoking, reduce alcohol intake, optimize glycaemic control
Medical: diuretics, ACE inhibitors, angiotensin receptor antagonists, calcium channel blockers, β-blockers

Cx Atherosclerosis, heart failure, cerebral infarct, cerebral haemorrhage, renal impairment

MALIGNANT HYPERTENSION

This is a **medical emergency**.

P Fibrinoid necrosis of small arteries/arterioles and dilatation of cerebral arteries

A ♂ > ♀; usually in 5th decade

S Headache, vomiting, visual disturbance, convulsions, papilloedema

Rx Intravenous labetalol/GTN, bring blood pressure (BP) down slowly

Cx Microangiopathic haemolytic anaemia, renal failure, cerebral haemorrhage, coma, death

ARRHYTHMIAS

ATRIAL FIBRILLATION (AF)

P Disorganized atrial activity, resulting in an irregular ventricular response

A See Box 1.3.

Box 1.3 CAUSES OF ATRIAL FIBRILLATION

- Ischaemic heart disease
- Lung disease
- Hypoxia
- Hypertension
- Rheumatic heart disease
- Sepsis
- Hypercapnia
- Alcohol
- Mitral stenosis
- Atrial septal defect
- Metabolic abnormalities
- Thyrotoxicosis

Sy Palpitations

Si Irregularly irregular pulse, with or without haemodynamic compromise

Ix ECG, investigations into the underlying cause

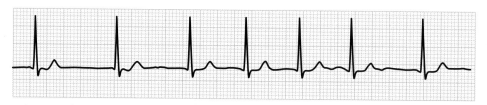

Figure 1.1 Atrial fibrillation: note the absence of P waves and irregularly irregular rhythm

Treatment of underlying cause; rate control (digoxin, β-blockers, diltiazem), anti-arrhythmics (amiodarone, flecainide), anticoagulation (warfarin/heparin), DC cardioversion to return to sinus rhythm

Cx Systemic embolization, rapid ventricular rate leading to hypotension/angina/heart failure

ATRIAL FLUTTER

P Atrial re-entry tachycardia, leading to rapid atrial rate (~300 beats/min); usually occurs with slower ventricular rate due to 2:1 or 3:1 block in the atrioventricular (AV) node

A Acute cardiac or respiratory problems e.g. pericarditis, pneumonia

Sy Palpitations

Si Tachycardia, with or without haemodynamic compromise

Ix ECG: usually reveals characteristic saw-tooth pattern with AV block

Rx *Rate control*: anti-arrhythmics, anticoagulation
Curative: DC cardioversion, catheter ablation of aberrant pathway

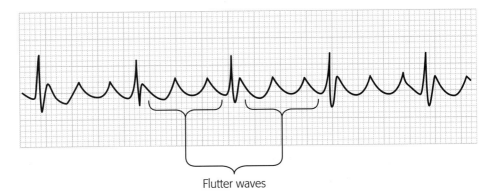

Flutter waves

Figure 1.2 Atrial flutter: note the characteristic 'F' waves

WOLFF–PARKINSON–WHITE SYNDROME (WPW)

P Atrial re-entry tachycardia, with an accessory excitatory pathway linking the atrium to the ventricle (bundle of Kent)

A Idiopathic

Sy Palpitations

Si Tachycardia

Ix ECG: short PR interval, delta wave (slurred upstroke to QRS), wide QRS

Rx DC cardioversion, β-blockers, calcium-channel blockers, catheter ablation

Cx Rarely may progress to ventricular fibrillation (VF)

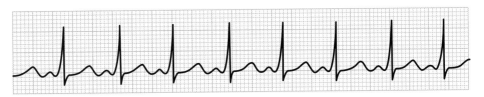

Figure 1.3 Wolff–Parkinson–White syndrome: note the short PR interval and slurred upstroke to the QRS complex

VENTRICULAR TACHYCARDIA (VT)

(P) *Sustained* VT is VT that lasts for >30 s or causes haemodynamic compromise

(A) Most commonly due to ischaemic heart disease ± MI; cardiomyopathy, metabolic abnormalities, drug toxicity, long QT syndrome

(Sy) Palpitations, chest pain, syncope

(Si) Tachycardia with hypotension, varying 1st heart sound, occasional cannon waves (giant 'a' waves in JVP)

(Ix) ECG (wide complex tachycardia)

(Rx) Anti-arrhythmics (amiodarone, lidocaine), DC cardioversion, implantable cardiac defibrillator to treat recurrence

(Cx) VF

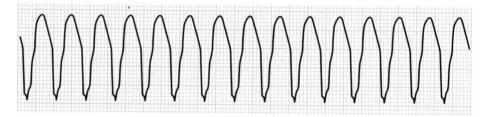

Figure 1.4 Ventricular tachycardia

VENTRICULAR FIBRILLATION

(A) Ischaemic heart disease, post-infarction, *torsades de pointes*, prolonged QT interval, severe hypoxia; VT can always degenerate into VF

(S) Syncope, cardiac arrest

(Ix) ECG/heart monitor

(Rx) DC cardioversion, anti-arrhythmics, intravenous magnesium, cardiac pacing, implanted cardiac defibrillator

(Cx) Death

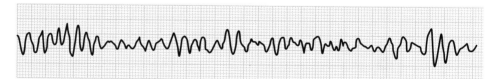

Figure 1.5 Ventricular fibrillation

ATRIOVENTRICULAR BLOCK (AVB)

(P) Due to damage to the atrial node, AV node or His/Purkinje system

(A) Myocardial infarction, drugs (digitalis, calcium channel blockers, β-blockers), myocarditis, acute rheumatic fever, sarcoid, infections (e.g. Lyme disease)

Box 1.4 CLASSIFICATION OF AV BLOCK

- *1st degree AVB*: PR interval >0.20 s (five small squares on ECG)
- *2nd degree AVB*: some atrial impulses fail to conduct to the ventricles
  - *Mobitz Type I* (Wenckebach): the PR interval gradually increases in length until there is a 'missed beat'
  - *Mobitz Type II*: occasional dropped QRS complexes are not related to changes in the PR interval
- *3rd degree AVB*: atrial and ventricular impulses are completely dissociated

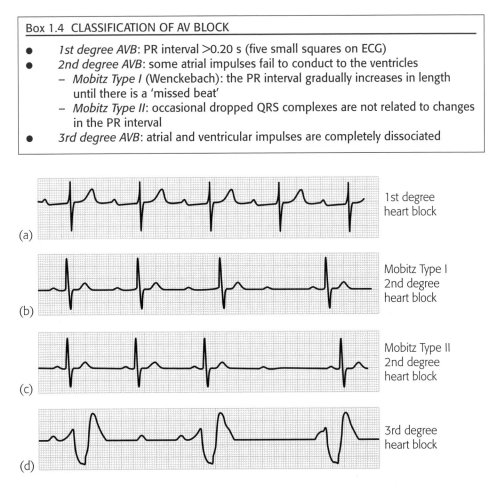

(a) 1st degree heart block

(b) Mobitz Type I 2nd degree heart block

(c) Mobitz Type II 2nd degree heart block

(d) 3rd degree heart block

Figure 1.6 (a) 1st degree heart block: prolonged PR interval; (b) Mobitz Type I 2nd degree heart block: progressive PR elongation; (c) Mobitz Type II 2nd degree heart block: fixed PR interval, with occasional P waves not being conducted to the ventricles; (d) 3rd degree AV block, there is no relationship between atrial and ventricular activity. The wide QRS complex is the result of a spontaneous escape rhythm of 35–40 beats/min

- **S** Syncope, dyspnoea, heart failure
- **Ix** ECG, cardiac monitoring
- **Rx** Atropine, isoprenaline (β-agonist); any patients with symptomatic 2nd or 3rd degree heart block should have cardiac pacing

VALVULAR HEART DISEASE

AORTIC STENOSIS

(P) A pressure gradient between the LV and aorta >50mmHg or aortic orifice <1 cm^2 leads to LV outflow obstruction: response is LV dilatation, muscle hypertrophy and ↓ stroke volume; hypertrophy leads to ↑ oxygen demand

(A) Degenerative calcification, rheumatic fever, congenital bicuspid valve

(Sy) Exertional dyspnoea, angina, heart failure, syncope, sudden death

(Si) Narrow pulse pressure, slow rising pulse, heaving apex beat, displaced apex beat, systolic thrill, ejection systolic murmur (heard best over the aortic valve in expiration ± radiation to the carotids), soft S2, paradoxical splitting of S2, 4th heart sound

(Ix) ECG (LV hypertrophy and 'strain'), CXR (LV enlargement, pulmonary congestion), echo, cardiac catheterization

(Rx) *Medical:* treatment aimed at symptoms (diuretics, nitrates, β-blockers)
Surgery: aortic valve replacement

AORTIC REGURGITATION

(P) Regurgitation leads to an increase in LV end-diastolic pressure, which leads to LV dilatation and hypertrophy

(A) Rheumatic fever, endocarditis, hypertension, atherosclerosis, Marfan's syndrome, syphilis, seronegative arthritis, aortic dissection

(Sy) Dyspnoea, arrhythmias, orthopnoea, paroxysmal nocturnal dyspnoea, angina

(Si) Heaving displaced apex beat, diastolic thrill, 3rd heart sound

---

Box 1.5 SIGNS OF AORTIC REGURGITATION

- Wide pulse pressure
- Large volume collapsing 'waterhammer' pulse
- Early diastolic, high-pitched murmur (heard best at lower left sternal edge, patient sitting forward)
- Visible carotid pulsations: Corrigan's sign
- Capillary pulsations in the nail bed: Quincke's sign
- 'Pistol shots' over the femoral arteries: Traube's sign
- Head nodding in time with the pulse: de Musset's sign
- Mid-diastolic murmur heard at the apex: Austin Flint murmur

---

(Ix) ECG (LV hypertrophy and strain, left axis deviation), echo, CXR (LV enlargement), cardiac catheterization

(Rx) *Medical:* treatment aimed at symptoms (diuretics, ACE inhibitors, vasodilators); nifedipine/ACE inhibitors may delay the need for surgery
Surgery: aortic valve replacement

MITRAL STENOSIS

(P) When the mitral valve orifice is <2 cm^2, the left atrium (LA) requires abnormally high pressures to propel blood into the LV and maintain cardiac output; this leads to a high AV pressure gradient; backward transmission of the high LA pressure leads to pulmonary hypertension

- **A** ♀ > ♂; rheumatic heart disease, congenital, endocarditis, systemic lupus erythematosus
- **Sy** Dyspnoea, orthopnoea, paroxysmal nocturnal dyspnoea, palpitations, right-sided heart failure
- **Si** Malar flush, atrial fibrillation, pulmonary oedema, ↑JVP with prominent a waves, tapping apex beat, left parasternal heave, loud 1st heart sound, opening snap, rumbling mid-diastolic murmur (accentuated with exertion, heard with patient on left side), stigmata of systemic embolization, may develop tricuspid regurgitation
- **Ix** ECG (tall P waves in V_1 and II; right axis deviation and RV hypertrophy in pulmonary hypertension; AF), echo, CXR (straightening of left border of heart, prominent pulmonary arteries), cardiac catheterization
- **Rx** *Medical*: treatment aimed at symptoms (diuretics, digoxin, β-blockers), warfarin (history of AF or systemic emboli)
  Surgery: mitral valvotomy (percutaneous balloon or surgical), mitral valve replacement

MITRAL REGURGITATION (MR)

- **P** Increasing regurgitant jet leads to an increase in LV volume and reduction in cardiac output
- **A** Rheumatic heart disease, ischaemic heart disease, post-infarction, hypertrophic cardiomyopathy, degenerative calcification, infective endocarditis, mitral valve prolapse, LV dilatation, connective tissue disorders
- **Sy** Dyspnoea, fatigue, orthopnoea, right-sided heart failure
- **Si** Jerky pulse, soft 1st heart sound, displaced apex beat, apical thrill, 3rd heart sound, pansystolic murmur, pulmonary oedema
- **Ix** ECG (LA ± RA may be enlarged), CXR (LA may be massively enlarged; ± pulmonary oedema), echo, cardiac catheterization
- **Rx** *Medical*: treatment aimed at symptoms (diuretics, ACE inhibitors, digoxin)
  Surgery: mitral valve replacement

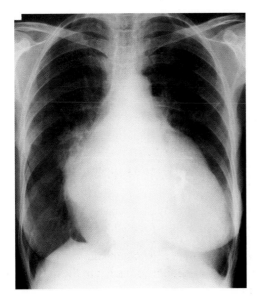

Figure 1.7 Mitral valve disease: enlarged heart with a double contour to the right cardiac border, indicating left atrial enlargement. Prominence of the left cardiac border is from the atrial appendage. Note the calcification in the mitral annulus

MITRAL VALVE PROLAPSE

(P) myxomatous degeneration

(A) ♀ > ♂; idiopathic, rheumatic heart disease, ischaemic heart disease, cardiomyopathy, connective tissue disorders e.g. Marfan's syndrome, Ehlers–Danlos syndrome

(Sy) May be asymptomatic; palpitations, syncope, chest pain, sudden death (rare)

(Si) Arrhythmias, mid-late systolic click, high pitched late-systolic murmur

(Ix) ECG, echo

(Rx) *Medical*: aimed at symptoms: anti-arrhythmics, antibiotic prophylaxis, β-blockers for chest pain
Surgery: Mitral valve repair/replacement if MR is a problem

(Cx) MR, infective endocarditis

PULMONARY STENOSIS

(P) Outflow obstruction may be valvular, subvalvular or supravalvular; transvalvular gradient grades the severity: <50 mmHg: mild; 50–80 mmHg: moderate; >80 mmHg: severe

(A) Congenital, associated with carcinoid syndrome

(Sy) Asymptomatic; fatigue, dyspnoea, syncope, symptoms associated with heart failure

(Si) *a* wave in the JVP, soft P2, 4th heart sound, left parasternal heave, thrill and ejection systolic murmur (left upper sternal border), increasing severity leads to a longer murmur,

(Ix) ECG (right axis deviation and RV hypertrophy), CXR (large left atrium), echo

(Rx) Balloon valvuloplasty; valve replacement rarely indicated

TRICUSPID REGURGITATION

(P) Usually functional: due to dilatation of the tricuspid annulus following right ventricular dilatation

(A) Functional (pulmonary hypertension, CCF, cardiomyopathy), rheumatic, tricuspid valve endocarditis, carcinoid, trauma, post-infarction, endomyocardial fibrosis

(Sy) Clinical features are due to venous congestion and reduced cardiac output

(Si) ↑JVP with prominent v waves, pansystolic murmur heard best at left lower sternal edge, pulsatile hepatomegaly, peripheral oedema, ascites, dyspnoea

(Ix) ECG, CXR (enlarged RA and RV), echo

(Rx) Aimed at underlying cause or surgery

CONGENITAL HEART DISEASE

ATRIAL SEPTAL DEFECT

(P) *Ostium primum*: septal defect lies adjacent to AV valve
Ostium secundum: mid-septum; 70 per cent of cases
Sinus venosus: high in septum, near superior vena cava (SVC)

(A) Congenital; ♀ > ♂; Down syndrome associated with ostium primum

(Sy) Usually asymptomatic until adulthood; palpitations (arrhythmias), dyspnoea, cyanosis

Si Left parasternal heave, wide fixed splitting of 2nd heart sound, mid-systolic murmur at left sternal edge (due to increased flow across the pulmonary valve), cyanosis, clubbing, occasional mid-diastolic murmur

Ix ECG (ostium primum: left axis deviation, ostium secundum: right axis deviation, right bundle branch block (RBBB); RV or RA hypertrophy), CXR (large hilar arteries, enlarged RV and RA, increased pulmonary vasculature), echo

Rx Small atrial septal defect (ASD) with minimum left-to-right shunts can be left; surgical closure

Cx Arrhythmias

VENTRICULAR SEPTAL DEFECT

P Usually in the membranous portion of the septum

A Congenital, post-infarction; commonest congenital anomaly; incidence ~0.2 per cent births; associated with Fallot's tetralogy

Sy Usually develop with reversal of the shunt; dyspnoea, chest pain, syncope, haemoptysis

Si Cyanosis, clubbing, loud pansystolic murmur

Ix Echo

Rx Spontaneous closure occurs in ~50 per cent small ventricular septal defects (VSDs); surgical correction when there is a moderate/large left-to-right shunt

Cx Congestive cardiac failure (CCF), pulmonary hypertension and reversal of shunt, RV outflow tract obstruction, aortic regurgitation, infective endocarditis

INFECTIVE/INFLAMMATORY CONDITIONS

PERICARDITIS

P Inflammation of the pericardium

A Viral, post-MI, uraemia, tuberculosis, rheumatic fever, connective tissue disorders, malignancy

Sy Substernal sharp chest pain, worse on movement and inspiration; relieved by sitting forward and worse on lying flat

Si Pericardial friction rub, fever

Ix ECG (widespread ST elevation, concave in shape, followed by T wave inversion)

Rx Non-steroidal anti-inflammatory drugs (NSAIDs) for pain; treatment of underlying condition

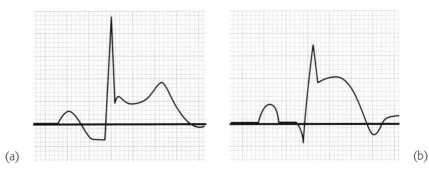

(a)   (b)

Figure 1.8 (a) Pericarditis. Note the concave ST elevation, compared with myocardial infarction (b)

MYOCARDITIS

(A) Infection, drugs, radiation; commonest cause is viruses – *Coxsackie*

(Sy) Variable; may be asymptomatic, chest pain, heart failure, palpitations, death

(Si) Often normal; occasionally 3rd heart sound, pansystolic murmur (MR)

(Ix) ECG (T wave or ST changes), viral screen (stool samples, throat swab, nasopharyngeal washings etc.), cardiac enzymes, echo

(Rx) Usually self-limiting; treatment aimed at symptoms/complications; patients rarely require intensive therapy unit (ITU)/cardiac transplantation

(Cx) Chronic myocarditis, dilated cardiomyopathy, heart failure

INFECTIVE ENDOCARDITIS

(P) Infection of the endothelium; usually involves the valves; vegetations are a mixture of bacteria, fibrin and platelets

(A) Intravenous drug use (IVDU), prosthetic valves, sporadic
Bacteria involved: ~10 per cent no causative organism, *Staphylococcus aureus* (IVDU), *Streptococci*, *Enterococci*, Gram-negative bacteria, *Candida*

(Sy) Separated into acute endocarditis (AE), a rapidly progressive illness, and subacute bacterial endocarditis (SBE), a slowly progressive condition
Fever, anorexia, weight loss, myalgia

(Si) See Box 1.6

Box 1.6 DIAGNOSIS OF ENDOCARDITIS

Duke Criteria: 2 major, 1 major + 3 minor, or 5 minor for diagnosis
- *Major*:
  - blood culture positive for typical organism or persistently positive
  - evidence of endocardial involvement
- *Minor*:
  - fever
  - previous heart condition or IVDU
  - immunological phenomena (due to immune complex deposition): Osler's nodes (raised tender nodules on finger pulps), Roth spots (small retinal haemorrhages), glomerulonephritis, clubbing, petechiae, arthralgia
  - vascular phenomena: mycotic aneurysms, Janeway lesions (painless macules on palm), septic emboli, intracranial haemorrhage, visceral infarct, splinter haemorrhages
  - positive blood culture with atypical bacteria

(Ix) FBC, C-reactive protein (CRP), erythrocyte sedimentation rate (ESR), blood cultures (minimum of 3), rheumatoid factor, immune complex titre, ECG, echo (trans-oesophageal echo is more sensitive)

(Rx) Broad-spectrum intravenous antibiotics until culture results available (check hospital policy, but usually i.v. benzylpenicillin + gentamicin); add flucloxacillin in IVDUs

(Cx) Septic emboli, mycotic aneurysms, meningitis, intracranial haemorrhage, emboli, glomerulonephritis

MISCELLANEOUS

HYPERTROPHIC OBSTRUCTIVE CARDIOMYOPATHY (HOCM)

P   Left ventricular hypertrophy, especially involving the septum; varying degrees of myocardial fibrosis

A   ~50 per cent patients have a +ve family history; multiple mutations have been identified; associated with Friedrich's ataxia

Sy   Many are asymptomatic; dyspnoea, fatigue, palpitations, angina, syncope, sudden death

Si   *a* wave in the JVP, double apical impulse, ejection systolic murmur at lower left sternal border, pansystolic murmur at the apex, 4th heart sound

Ix   ECG (LV hypertrophy, Q waves, arrhythmias), CXR (increased cardiothoracic ratio [CTR]), echo (asymmetric septal hypertrophy, systolic anterior motion of the mitral valve, small LV cavity with posterior wall motion, MR)

Rx   β-blockers/verapamil to improve LV function, amiodarone as anti-arrhythmic, surgery (myotomy/myectomy), ethanol injections into the septum (causes partial infarction of the septum), cardiac pacing; avoidance of any drugs that significantly lower the preload

Cx   Arrhythmias, ischaemia, sudden death

ATRIAL MYXOMA

P   Benign tumour; gelatinous polypoid structure attached to the atrial septum; usually left atrium

A   ♀ > ♂; 3rd–6th decades; most are sporadic; occasionally familial (autosomal dominant)

Sy   Fever, dyspnoea, weight loss, arthralgia, syncope; can mimic mitral valve disease (stenosis from the tumour prolapsing into the valve, or regurgitation from related valve trauma)

Si   Loud 1st heart sound, tumour 'plop' (a loud 3rd heart sound), clubbing

Ix   Echo, FBC (anaemia or polycythaemia), ↑ESR

Rx   Surgical resection

Cx   Peripheral or pulmonary emboli

RESPIRATORY

RESPIRATORY INVESTIGATIONS

- **Chest radiography (CXR):** be careful to look at the apices, behind the heart and costophrenic angles
- **Computed tomography (CT):** better at distinguishing between tissue densities and assessing lesions; high-resolution CT shows subtle parenchymal changes; CT pulmonary angiography (CTPA) can diagnose pulmonary emboli in the segmental and larger pulmonary arteries
- **Ventilation–perfusion scans:** albumin labelled with technetium 99m is administered intravenously to demonstrate blood flow, and radiolabelled xenon gas is inhaled to demonstrate ventilation. This shows mismatches in ventilation and perfusion, and is commonly used to diagnose pulmonary embolism.
- **Positron emission tomography (PET):** used to identify malignant lesions and stage lung cancer. A radiolabelled glucose analogue is injected and is taken up by metabolically active malignant cells.
- **Arterial blood gases:** for interpretation see 'Respiratory failure' section (p. 15)
- **PEFR (peak expiratory flow rate):** useful in asthma
- **Spirometry:** measures inspired and expired gas volume against time:
  - FEV_1 – forced expiratory volume in 1 second
  - FVC – forced vital capacity (total volume exhaled)
  $$\frac{FEV_1}{FVC}:$$
  normal range 0.75–0.80
  <0.75 = obstructive defect
  >0.80 = restrictive defect
- **Sputum:** microscopy, culture, Gram stain, cytology and sensitivities.
- **Bronchoscopy:** allowing direct visualization of the bronchial tree. Samples can be taken by biopsy, brushings or broncho-alveolar lavage (BAL).
- **Video-assisted thoracic surgery (VATS):** a rigid endoscope is passed into the pleura to allow visualization and biopsy of pleural or parenchymal disease.

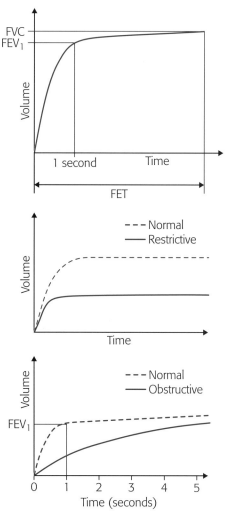

Figure 1.9 Interpretation of spirometry results (adapted with kind permission from Dakin J, Kourteli E and Winter R, *Making Sense of Lung Function Tests A Hands-on Guide*, Great Britain: Arnold, 2003)

RESPIRATORY FAILURE

 Respiration requires the integrated function of the nervous system, airways, alveoli, musculature and vasculature. Failure of any of these can lead to respiratory failure:
- Type I respiratory failure: hypoxia with normal partial pressure of carbon dioxide (P_{CO_2})
- Type II respiratory failure: hypoxia and hypercapnia

(A) See Fig. 1.10

Hypoxaemia has four causes:
- hypoventilation
- ventilation–perfusion ($\dot{V}/\dot{Q}$) mismatch
- shunting
- ↓ in inspired partial pressure of oxygen (P_{O_2})

(Rx) Management is aimed at the underlying cause:
- initial treatment is to administer high-flow oxygen
- patients may require assisted ventilation; this can be given as non-invasive positive pressure ventilation (NIPPV) – this can eliminate CO_2 (and hence acidosis)
- if this fails they will require mechanical ventilation

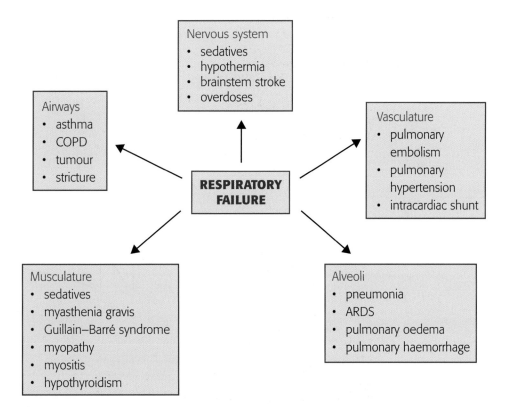

Figure 1.10 Respiratory failure
ARDS: acute respiratory distress syndrome; COPD: chronic obstructive pulmonary disease

AIRWAYS DISEASE

ASTHMA[1]

P Chronic reversible inflammation of the airways caused by increased sensitivity to various stimuli; leading to variable airway obstruction

A Atopy, family history (especially maternal), parental smoking increases the risk of childhood asthma

Triggers: dust, emotion, exercise, cold weather, NSAID/β-blockers etc.

Sy None when well

Wheeze, cough, dyspnoea, chest tightness, night-time waking

Si None when well

Tachypnoea, tachycardia, cyanosis, wheeze

Diurnal variation

Ix *PEFR* (peak expiratory flow rate) *and spirometry:* expected >25 per cent variability

CXR: if any atypical symptoms or exacerbations (to rule out pneumothorax/infection etc.)

Rx Avoidance of pollutants/allergens/smoking; weight loss in obesity

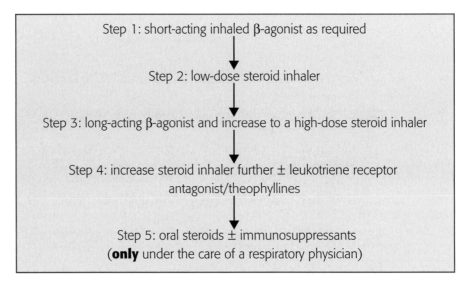

Step 1: short-acting inhaled β-agonist as required

Step 2: low-dose steroid inhaler

Step 3: long-acting β-agonist and increase to a high-dose steroid inhaler

Step 4: increase steroid inhaler further ± leukotriene receptor antagonist/theophyllines

Step 5: oral steroids ± immunosuppressants
(**only** under the care of a respiratory physician)

Figure 1.11 Management of chronic asthma

NB:

1   beware the side-effects of long-term steroids: osteoporosis, diabetes mellitus, hypertension, easy bruising (see Cushing's syndrome p. 66)

2   check inhaler technique – need for a spacer device?

Acute asthma

This is a **medical emergency**.

Box 1.7 CLASSIFICATION OF ACUTE ASTHMA

- **Moderate exacerbation**
  - PEFR 50–75% predicted/best
  - Worsening symptoms
- **Severe asthma**
  - PEFR 33–50% predicted/best
  - Unable to complete sentences in one breath
  - Exhaustion/poor respiratory effort
  - Tachycardia (HR >110 beats/min)
  - Tachypnoea (RR >25 breaths/min)
- **Life-threatening asthma**
  - Silent chest
  - Po_2 <8 kPa
  - Normal or rising Pco_2
  - Bradycardia
  - Hypotension
  - Confusion

HR: heart rate
RR: respiration rate

Ix Pulse oximetry, PEFR, arterial blood gases if saturations are <92 per cent
CXR **only** if signs of pneumothorax/consolidation/failure to respond/life-threatening asthma

Rx High-flow oxygen, nebulized beta agonist bronchodilators, nebulized ipratropium bromide, oral steroids
If no improvement: magnesium sulphate infusion ± aminophylline infusion
Call for help early
The patient should be closely monitored with pulse oximetry and PEFR

CHRONIC OBSTRUCTIVE PULMONARY DISEASE (COPD)/EMPHYSEMA

P Chronic inflammatory condition which causes progressive airflow obstruction secondary to parenchymal damage

A Smoking, α_1-antitrypsin deficiency

S Breathlessness, cough, sputum production, wheeze
Signs of cor pulmonale (see p. 28)
Very little diurnal variation in symptoms, and less reversibility than asthma (<20 per cent)

Ix CXR, FBC, BMI (body mass index), ECG, theophylline level (if applicable)
Spirometry: FEV_1 <80 per cent predicted, $\frac{FEV_1}{FVC}$ <0.7 (obstructive picture)

Rx *Acute exacerbation*:
- oxygen – beware Type II respiratory failure!
- nebulizers (β_2-agonists/anticholinergics)
- steroids
- aminophylline infusions
- NIPPV

Chronic:
- – smoking cessation
- – vaccinations
- – pulmonary rehabilitation
- – surgery

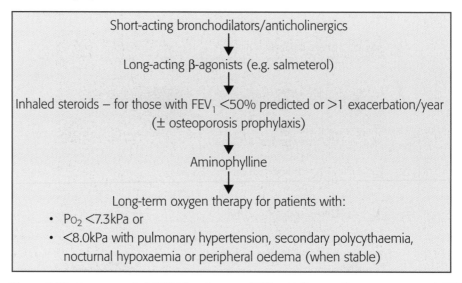

Short-acting bronchodilators/anticholinergics

↓

Long-acting β-agonists (e.g. salmeterol)

↓

Inhaled steroids – for those with FEV_1 <50% predicted or >1 exacerbation/year
(± osteoporosis prophylaxis)

↓

Aminophylline

↓

Long-term oxygen therapy for patients with:
- • Po_2 <7.3kPa or
- • <8.0kPa with pulmonary hypertension, secondary polycythaemia,
  nocturnal hypoxaemia or peripheral oedema (when stable)

Figure 1.12 Management of COPD/emphysema ('BTS guidelines on the management of COPD',
Thorax 1997;52, Supplement V, adapted with kind permission from BMJ Publishing Group)

α_1-ANTITRYPSIN DEFICIENCY

P   Lack of α_1-antitrypsin, an enzyme made in the liver, that controls the breakdown of other enzymes in the body

A   Autosomal recessive disease; affects all populations

S   All symptoms related to emphysema and cirrhosis; onset of these conditions at a younger age, with no other causes

Ix   As for emphysema and cirrhosis; serum α_1-antitrypsin levels can be measured

Rx   As for emphysema and cirrhosis; liver ± lung transplantation

INFECTIONS[2]

COMMUNITY-ACQUIRED PNEUMONIA

P   Commonly *S. pneumoniae*; *Legionella* and *Staphylococcus* are more common in patients admitted to ITU; 'atypical' bacteria include *Chlamydia pneumoniae, Mycoplasma pneumoniae, Chlamydia psittaci, Coxiella burnetii*

A   Mortality 4–10 per cent; increased incidence in the elderly, COPD, diabetes, alcoholics, nursing home residents
Epidemics of *Mycoplasma pneumoniae* occur every 4 years in the UK; *Legionella* infection may occur more often in young people and those exposed to poorly maintained air conditioning systems
Staphylococcus is related to the influenza virus

Sy Cough, fever, dyspnoea, tachypnoea, pleuritic pain, myalgia

'Atypical' pneumonias may present with diarrhoea or abdominal pain

Si Crepitations, bronchial breathing, hypoxia/cyanosis

Ix CXR, FBC, U&E, CRP, LFT, sputum culture and Gram stain

In severe community-acquired pneumonia: viral and 'atypical' pathogen serology, pneumococcal and *Legionella* urine antigen detection, blood cultures

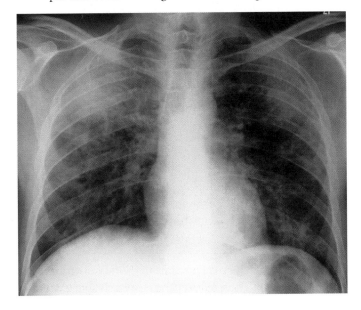

Figure 1.13 Bilateral patchy shadowing throughout both lungfields – bronchopneumonia

---

Box 1.8 CURB-65 SCORE

This is a 6-point score system to assess severity of community acquired pneumonia on presentation to hospital

One point for each of the following:

- **C**onfusion
- **U**rea >7 mmol/L
- **R**espiratory rate >30/min
- systolic **B**lood pressure <90 mmHg
- diastolic **B**lood pressure <60 mmHg
- age >**65** years

CURB score 0: low risk of death; no need for hospital admission

CURB score 1–2: increased risk of death; should be admitted

CURB score 3 or more: high risk of death; urgent hospital admission

Source: Lim WS, van der Eerden MM, Laing R *et al*. Defining community acquired pneumonia severity on presentation to hospital: an international derivation and validation study. *Thorax* 2003;58:377–82.

Rx *Non-severe*: amoxicillin + erythromycin/clarithromycin (fluoroquinolone if penicillin allergic)

Severe: co-amoxiclav/cefuroxime/3rd generation cephalosporin + erythromycin/clarithromycin

Saline nebulizers may aid expectoration

Intravenous fluids if there are any signs of dehydration/renal impairment

PULMONARY TUBERCULOSIS

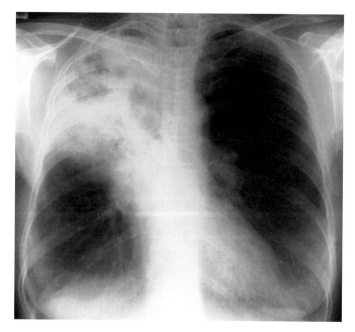

Figure 1.14 Cavitating consolidation in the right upper lobe – active tuberculosis

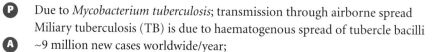 Due to *Mycobacterium tuberculosis*; transmission through airborne spread
Miliary tuberculosis (TB) is due to haematogenous spread of tubercle bacilli

A ~9 million new cases worldwide/year;
↑incidence in the UK through the 1990s due to HIV infection, immigration from countries with high prevalence, social problems/homelessness

Sy Can have an acute (often in the young or immunocompromised) or insidious onset
Tachypnoea, cough, haemoptysis, lethargy, weakness, weight loss, anorexia, night sweats, fever

Si Often no findings on chest examination; crepitations in upper zones, lymphadenopathy

Ix Sputum microscopy and culture for AFB (acid-fast bacilli), CXR, Mantoux
If diagnosis is difficult consider bronchoscopy and biopsy/brushings/broncho-alveolar lavage (BAL)

Rx 6 month regime: 2 months of *RIPE*:
- Rifampicin,
- Isoniazid,
- Pyrazinamide,
- Ethambutol

followed by rifampicin and isoniazid for 4 months
Multi-drug-resistant TB (MDR-TB): defined as resistance to rifampicin and isoniazid; treatment is complicated and must be done under specialist centres, usually involving five or more drugs to which the bacteria is susceptible for a minimum of 9 months (and often much longer)

Cx All anti-TB drugs have serious side-effects:
– pyridoxine is given to prevent peripheral neuropathy from isoniazid

 – prior to starting treatment visual acuity should be assessed and renal/liver
   function monitored throughout
All cases of TB should be notified to the local consultant in communicable disease
control
Contact tracing should be performed

PLEURAL DISEASE[3]

PLEURAL EFFUSION

 Transudate (protein <25 g/L): heart failure, hypoalbuminaemia, cirrhosis,
hypothyroidism, peritoneal dialysis, PE
Exudate (protein >35 g/L): carcinoma, pneumonia, TB, rheumatoid arthritis,
systemic lupus erythematosus (SLE), lymphoma, mesothelioma, pancreatitis, drugs
(amiodarone, nitrofurantoin, methotrexate)
An **empyema** refers to a grossly purulent pleural effusion

 Breathlessness

Tracheal deviation, decreased expansion, stony dull percussion note, diminished
breath sounds

Imaging: CXR, bronchoscopy and high-resolution CT (HRCT) scan may be required
to determine the underlying cause
Pleural aspirate: for protein, microscopy, Gram stain, culture, cytology, glucose,
lactate dehydrogenase (LDH), pH, acid- and alcohol-fast bacilli (AAFB) culture ±
amylase/triglycerides

Box 1.9 LIGHT'S CRITERIA FOR PLEURAL EFFUSIONS

For pleural protein 25–35 g/L; the fluid is an exudate if:
- pleural fluid protein divided by serum protein > 0.5
- pleural fluid LDH divided by serum LDH > 0.6
- pleural fluid LDH > two-thirds the upper limit of normal serum LDH.

Source: Light RW, Macgregor MI, Luchsinger PC, Ball WC Jr. Pleural effusions: the
diagnostic separation of transudates and exudates. *Annals of Internal Medicine*
1972;77:507–13.

---

pH: normal ~7.6; drainage required if pH <7.2 in an infected effusion
Glucose: low in empyema, rheumatoid, lupus, TB, malignancy
Amylase: raised in acute pancreatitis, oesophageal rupture, malignancy
Cytology: positive in ~60 per cent malignancy

 Aimed at the underlying cause
If there is any respiratory compromise a pleurocentesis should be performed. If fluid
re-accumulates a chest drain should be considered

PARAPNEUMONIC EFFUSIONS

Pleural fluid will develop in 57 per cent of cases of pneumonia; in rarer cases there is
no obvious precipitant to the effusion
Commonest pathogens include *Streptococcus, Haemophilus influenzae, Escherichia
coli, Pseudomonas, Klebsiella*

(S) A combination of the symptoms and signs of pneumonia and pleural effusions

(Ix) As for pneumonia/pleural effusion

Ultrasound imaging can help with diagnosis

Pleural aspiration is *fundamental*

(Rx) Antibiotics

Chest drain is necessary if:
- pleural fluid pH <7.2
- pleural fluid glucose <2.2 mmol/L
- pleural LDH >1000 IU/L
- positive Gram stain/culture
- gross pus is aspirated (this is an empyema)

If the infection fails to resolve, refer to cardiothoracic surgery

SPONTANEOUS PNEUMOTHORAX

(P) Rupture of pleural bleb

(A) Commonest in young men ($\male$:$\female$ 6:1); COPD, asthma, carcinoma, cystic fibrosis, TB, connective tissue disorders

(Sy) Pleuritic pain, breathlessness

(Si) Tachycardia, tachypnoea, deviated trachea, diminished breath sounds, hyper-resonance, decreased vocal resonance

(Ix) CXR, CT scan if differentiating pneumothorax from bullous lung disease

(Rx) High-flow oxygen

Rim of air <2 cm and patient not breathless: discharge with early follow-up (if patient has underlying lung disease, observe for 24 h)

Rim of air >2 cm and breathless: aspirate

If patient is >50 years and has underlying lung disease: insertion of intercostal drain

If aspiration fails: insertion of intercostal drain

If lung fails to re-expand: refer to respiratory specialist to consider suction ± pleurodesis (artificial obliteration of the pleural space)

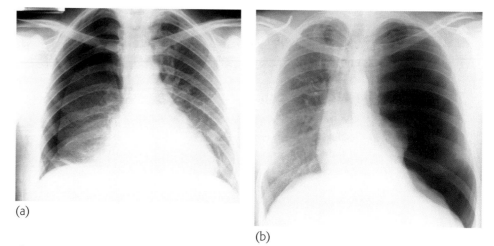

(a)

(b)

Figure 1.15 (a) Right pneumothorax: absence of lung markings beyond the lung edge; (b) left-sided tension pneumothorax. Note the mediastinal shift away from the affected side

Cx Tension pneumothorax – severe dyspnoea, hypotension, severe tachycardia, mediastinal shift

PULMONARY FIBROSIS[4]

A See Box 1.10

Box 1.10 CAUSES OF PULMONARY FIBROSIS

- *Occupation* (see below): exposure to pets/birds EAA (extrinsic allergic alveolitis)
- *Previous radiotherapy*
- *Drugs*: amiodarone, methotrexate, nitrofurantoin, penicillamine, bleomycin, cyclophosphamide
- *Systemic disorders*: vasculitis (Wegener's granulomatosis, Churg–Strauss syndrome, Behçet's syndrome, Goodpasture's syndrome, sarcoidosis)
- *Connective tissue disorders*: SLE, rheumatoid arthritis, Sjögren's syndrome, systemic sclerosis, polymyositis
- *Neoplasm*: lymphoma, lymphangitic carcinoma
- *Inherited disorders*: tuberous sclerosis, neurofibromatosis
- *Others*: amyloidosis

Sy Cough, shortness of breath, pleurisy more common in SLE/rheumatoid arthritis

Si Fine end-inspiratory crepitations, finger clubbing, weight loss, fatigue, hypoxaemia, signs of systemic disease

Ix *Bloods*: FBC, U&E, LFT, calcium levels, ACE (angiotensin-converting enzyme) levels
Immunology: anti-GBM (glomerular basement membrane), autoantibodies, ANA (antinuclear antibodies), ANCA (antineutrophil cytoplasmic antibodies), rheumatoid factor, serum precipitins
Imaging: CXR, HRCT
Spirometry: lung function tests: restrictive defect, reduced transfer factor, reduced lung volume
Endoscopy: bronchoscopy + BAL/biopsy

Rx Treatment for IPF (idiopathic pulmonary fibrosis), EAA, occupational lung disease and sarcoidosis is mentioned in each individual section
Treatment for fibrosis aimed at systemic/neoplastic conditions is aimed at the underlying condition

IDIOPATHIC PULMONARY FIBROSIS (IPF)

Previously known as cryptogenic fibrosing alveolitis (CFA)

(A)   Prevalence 6–15 per 100 000; incidence increases with age

(Si)   Bilateral fine end-inspiratory crepitations in 90 per cent of patients; finger clubbing in 50–70 per cent

(Rx)   Steroids and azathioprine; if azathioprine fails/is not tolerated cyclophosphamide

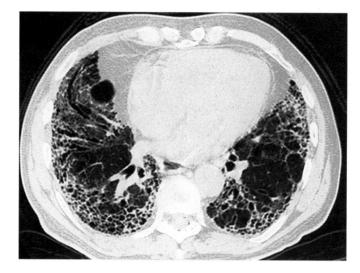

Figure 1.16 CT scan showing extensive interstitial thickening with small cystic spaces in a patient with idiopathic pulmonary fibrosis

EXTRINSIC ALLERGIC ALVEOLITIS (EAA)

(P)   Hypersensitivity reaction to various antigens

(A)   Less likely to be smokers than the general population
Farmer's lung (*Thermoactinomyces* in mouldy hay) and bird fancier's lung (avian protein on feathers) are most common; other antigens include isocyanates (chemical workers), *Aspergillus* spp. (tobacco workers)

(S)   Symptoms usually regress when the causative agent is removed

(Ix)   Serum precipitins to potential allergens e.g. *Micropolyspora faeni*, *Thermoactinomyces vulgaris*: eosinophilia is **not** a feature
CXR often shows apical sparing

(Rx)   Removal from exposure to the antigen; steroids speed up recovery

OCCUPATIONAL LUNG DISEASE

(A)   Asbestos, silica, cobalt, coal worker's pneumoconiosis, siderosis (iron), copper sulphate, aluminium, beryllium, cotton dust, grain dust

(S)   Variable, some dusts are more toxic/fibrogenic

(Rx)   Protective apparatus to prevent inhalation

ASBESTOSIS

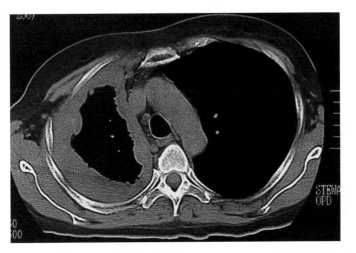

Figure 1.17
Mesothelioma: CT
showing extensive right-
sided pleural thickening

P Diffuse interstitial fibrosis
Usually manifests >10 years post-exposure
Pleural plaques indicate exposure to asbestos, not pulmonary involvement

A >80 per cent mesotheliomas are associated with asbestos exposure
Increased risk of lung cancer (squamous cell and adenocarcinoma)
Smoking increases the risk further, therefore patients should be advised to stop

Ix CXR may show fibrosis ± pleural plaques

Rx Palliation is the mainstay of treatment for mesothelioma

Px 50 per cent mesotheliomas metastasize, but most are locally invasive
Very poor prognosis

PULMONARY SARCOIDOSIS

P Chronic multisystem disorder which can affect any organ; accumulation of
granulomas and T lymphocytes

A Unknown cause; 75 per cent are aged 20–40 years, however it can affect all sexes,
ages, races and places of origin

S This depends on the organs involved
Pulmonary sarcoidosis can present subacutely or insidiously
Fever, malaise, weight loss, dyspnoea, cough
Combination of erythema nodosum and bilateral hilar lymphadenopathy is
pathognomonic

CXR shows abnormalities in 90 per cent

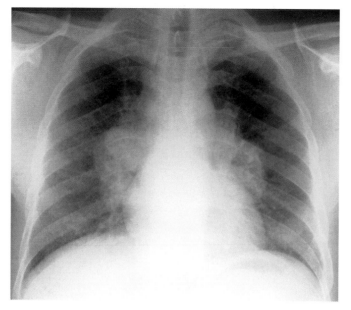

Figure 1.18 Bilateral hilar lymphadenopathy in sarcoidosis

Table 1.1 Chest X-ray grading in sarcoidosis

Grade	Abnormality
0	No abnormality
1	Lymphadenopathy alone
2	Lymphadenopathy and infiltrates
3	Infiltrates alone
4	Fibrosis

$\uparrow Ca^{2+}$, echocardiogram, $\uparrow$ serum ACE levels are poorly specific, but can be used to monitor disease activity

(Rx) Majority of patients do not need treatment

For persistent symptoms, steroids can be given and reduced slowly over months

For resistant disease consider methotrexate or chloroquine

SUPPURATIVE LUNG CONDITIONS

BRONCHIECTASIS

(P) Chronic inflammation and infection of the bronchial walls, leading to permanent dilatation of the airways

(A) Cystic fibrosis, pertussis, measles, TB, mechanical obstruction, Kartagener's syndrome (situs inversus and ciliary dysfunction), immunoglobulin deficiency

(Sy) Copious purulent sputum, recurrent chest infections

(Si) Clubbing, coarse inspiratory and expiratory crackles

(Ix) CXR, sputum culture, HRCT chest, immunoglobulins

(Rx) Postural drainage, antibiotics (commonest pathogens: *Staphylococcus aureus, Haemophilus influenzae, Pseudomonas aeruginosa*), bronchodilators, surgery

(Cx) Massive haemoptysis, cerebral abscess

CYSTIC FIBROSIS

 Autosomal recessive; abnormal chloride channels in the luminal surface lead to increased re-absorption of sodium and water leading to increased viscosity of airway secretions

 Recurrent childhood chest infections, failure to thrive, meconium ileus, steatorrhoea, bronchiectasis, male infertility, diabetes mellitus, gallstones

Clubbing, purulent sputum, central cyanosis, bilateral coarse crackles

Sweat testing, genetic testing, immunoreactive trypsin assay

Antibiotics, postural drainage, pancreatic supplements, low-fat diet, bronchodilators, heart–lung transplantation

MISCELLANEOUS

PULMONARY EMBOLISM

Immobility, trauma, recent surgery, pregnancy, malignancy, pro-thrombotic disorders, air travel, oral oestrogens

Dyspnoea, tachypnoea, pleuritic pain, haemoptysis, cough

Tachycardia, hypotension, ↑ JVP, clinical deep vein thrombosis (DVT)

Bloods: arterial blood gases, D-dimer (beware false positives),
ECG: S1Q3T3 pattern only seen in 10 per cent of PE
Imaging: CXR, V̇/Q̇ scan, CTPA, Doppler ultrasound scan (USS) leg, echo (only useful in massive central PE)

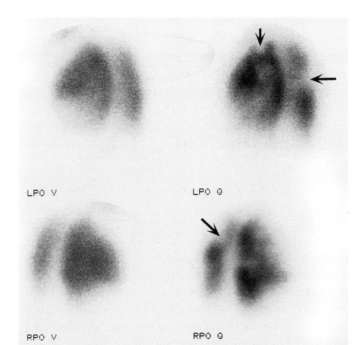

Figure 1.19 Isotope ventilation and perfusion scan: normal ventilation scan (V̇) but the perfusion (Q̇) scan shows multiple defects in pulmonary embolus

Rx   Oxygen, analgesia
Anticoagulation: usually with LMWH until PE confirmed, and then with warfarin
Thrombolysis: only in massive PE with haemodynamic compromise
Surgery: embolectomy, inferior vena cava (IVC) filters (to prevent recurrence)

PULMONARY HYPERTENSION/COR PULMONALE

P   Pulmonary hypertension (PH) refers to ↑ pulmonary artery pressure – it can be primary or secondary
Cor pulmonale refers to right ventricular enlargement secondary to pulmonary disease
Primary pulmonary hypertension (PPH): extremely rare
Secondary pulmonary hypertension: lung disease leads to increased pulmonary vascular resistance; to preserve cardiac output the right ventricle has to increase its output

Sy   Dyspnoea, fatigue, weakness, angina (RV [right ventricle] ischaemia), syncope

Si   ↑ JVP, peripheral oedema, loud P2, right-sided 4th heart sound, RV heave, tricuspid regurgitation, pulsatile hepatomegaly

Ix   Investigations to diagnose secondary causes of PH: CXR, ventilation-perfusion scan, HRCT, pulmonary function tests, lung biopsy, FBC (polycythaemia)
Investigations confirming PH: ECG (right axis deviation/RV hypertrophy), echocardiogram (RV and RA enlargement), cardiac catheterization (not usually necessary)

Rx   Treat the underlying cause; cor pulmonale is treated as for right heart failure (diuretics/oxygen)

BRONCHIAL CARCINOMA

P   Squamous cell 48 per cent, small cell (SCLC) 24 per cent, adenocarcinoma 13 per cent, large cell 10 per cent, other 5 per cent

A   Smoking (85 per cent), asbestos, nickel, air pollution
Commonest cancer of the Western world (and rapidly rising incidence in the developing world)

Sy   Cough, dyspnoea, haemoptysis, hoarse voice (laryngeal nerve invasion), weight loss

Si   Horner's syndrome (Pancoast's tumour), superior vena caval obstruction, lymphadenopathy, clubbing, hypertrophic pulmonary osteoarthropathy

---

Box 1.11 FEATURES OF HORNER'S SYNDROME

- Miosis (constricted pupil)
- Ptosis
- Anhidrosis (loss of sweating over half of face)
- Apparent enophthalmos

Ix   CXR, bronchoscopy + biopsy/brushings, sputum cytology, CT of the thorax/abdomen, lung function tests

Rx   *Surgery*: only possible if FEV_1 >1.5 L for lobectomy/>2 L for pneumonectomy
Radiotherapy (RT): radical RT for inoperable non-SCLC patients
Chemotherapy: first-line treatment for SCLC

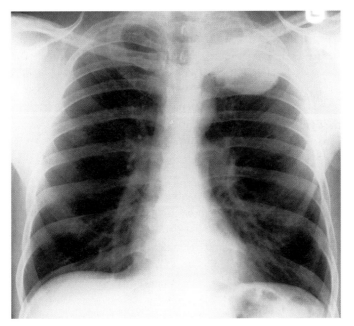

Figure 1.20 Pancoast's tumour at the left apex

REFERENCES

1   The British Thoracic Society/Scottish Intercollegiate Guidelines Network British Guideline on the Management of Asthma. *Thorax* 2003;58(Suppl I).
2   British Thoracic Society Guidelines for the Management of Community Acquired Pneumonia in Adults. *Thorax* 2001;56(Suppl IV) and 2004 Update.
3   British Thoracic Society Guidelines for the Management of Pleural Disease. *Thorax* 2003;58 (Suppl II).
4   British Thoracic Society and Standards of Care Committee. The diagnosis assessment and treatment of diffuse parenchymal lung disease in adults. *Thorax* 1999;54:1–28.

GASTROENTEROLOGY

GASTROINTESTINAL INVESTIGATIONS

- **Iron, folate, calcium:** absorbed in proximal small intestine
- **B_{12}:** absorbed in the terminal ileum
- **Endoscopy:**
    allows direct visualization of gastrointestinal (GI) tract and therapeutic procedures, OGD (oesophagogastroduodenoscopy)/jejunoscopy/sigmoidoscopy/colonoscopy therapies include variceal banding, injection of bleeding points with sclerosants, dilatation of strictures, stent placement
- **Barium studies:** allow visualization of GI mucosa
- **Urinary D-xylose test:** tests carbohydrate absorption; D-xylose is absorbed in proximal small intestine and excreted in the urine, therefore low excretion reflects poor absorption
- **Breath tests (BT):** commonly lactose–hydrogen BT (for lactose intolerance) or glucose–hydrogen BT (for bacterial overgrowth)
- **SeHCAT scan:** (selenium-75-homocholic acid taurine) nuclear medicine scan which assesses bile salt malabsorption; radiolabelled bile salts ingested, then scanned at 3 h and 7 days; if <15 per cent present at 7 days this suggests bile acid malabsorption
- **3-day faecal fat collection:** patient is given a high-fat diet during this test and every stool sample collected for 3 days; normal faecal fat is <18 mmol/day; increased in fat malabsorption or bile salt malabsorption
- **Faecal elastase:** reduced in chronic pancreatitis or pancreatic insufficiency
- **Pancreolauryl test:** test of pancreatic exocrine function

---

MALABSORPTION

P   Can be malabsorption of fat, carbohydrate, protein, vitamins or a combination of all

A   See Box 1.12

Box 1.12 CAUSES OF MALABSORPTION

- Coeliac disease
- Protein-losing enteropathy
- Whipple's disease
- Bacterial overgrowth
- Short bowel syndrome
- Tropical sprue
- Crohn's disease
- Lactose intolerance
- Chronic pancreatitis

History will give clues to potential diagnoses e.g. recent travel, recent bowel resection, dairy product intolerance, chronic pancreatitis etc.

Sy   Diarrhoea, steatorrhoea, weight loss

Si   Anaemia, oedema, hypovitaminosis

Ix   FBC, U&E, LFT, albumin, calcium, folate, iron, B_{12}, vitamin D, coagulation, coeliac serology, thyroid function[1]

Further investigations depend on history and results of blood tests indicating possible region of bowel involved:

- *Imaging*: OGD + small bowel biopsy, barium follow-through (BaFT), sigmoidoscopy/colonoscopy, barium enema, SeHCAT scan
- *Functional testing*: 24-h faecal fat, faecal elastase, urinary D-xylose test, 24-h urinary protein (if albumin low), gut hormones

 Rx aimed at underlying cause:
- *Whipple's disease/bacterial overgrowth/tropical sprue*: antibiotics
- *coeliac disease*: gluten-free diet
- *lactose intolerance*: avoidance of dairy products
- *short bowel syndrome*: anti-diarrhoeals, low-fat, high-fibre diet; nutritional replacement
- *chronic pancreatitis*: enzyme supplements

COELIAC DISEASE

P Gluten sensitivity leading to small intestinal enteropathy;

A Affects all ages; peak in 3rd decade

Sy Lethargy, weakness, diarrhoea, reduced fertility, weight loss

Si Anaemia

Ix *Diagnostic tests*: OGD + intestinal biopsy showing subtotal villous atrophy, coeliac antibodies (including antibodies to gliadin, endomysium and tissue transglutaminase [tTG])

Tests for malabsorption: FBC, iron, folate, B_{12}, albumin and calcium

Rx Gluten exclusion lifelong

Cx Small intestinal lymphoma/adenocarcinoma, osteopenia, dermatitis herpetiformis, hyposplenism

IRRITABLE BOWEL SYNDROME

P GI symptoms in the absence of structural pathology; abnormal autonomic reactivity, visceral hypersensitivity

A Post-infective, stress, adverse life events, psychological problems: anxiety, depression

Sy Abdominal discomfort, relief with defaecation, alternating bowel habit, bloating

Ix In a patient <45 years with a long history of typical symptoms, further investigations, beyond routine blood tests, should not be required

In a patient >45 years, with a short history or atypical symptoms, investigations should be done to exclude other pathologies – FBC, TFT, coeliac antibodies, inflammatory markers, sigmoidoscopy, diarrhoea/malabsorption screen

 Rx *Supportive*: explanation and reassurance, lifestyle advice

Medical: drug treatment is aimed at particular symptoms: antispasmodics (e.g. mebeverine), antidepressants, treatment for diarrhoea (loperamide, codeine), treatment for constipation, peppermint oil

Dietary: symptom diary to assess dietary factors, exclusion diets

Psychological: cognitive–behavioural therapy

INFLAMMATORY BOWEL DISEASE

CROHN'S DISEASE

(P) Affects any part of the GI tract from mouth to anus; segmental; transmural process; ulceration, cobblestone appearance, pseudopolyps, non-caseating granulomas, fissures, fistulae

(A) Genetic predisposition, smoking

(Sy) Depends on site affected; abdominal pain, diarrhoea, weight loss, per rectum (PR) mucus/pus, arthritis

(Si) Fever, malaise, anaemia, palpable inflammatory mass, fistulae, erythema nodosum, pyoderma gangrenosum

(Ix) Stool microscopy/culture, ↑ CRP, ↑ ESR, ↓ Hb, ↓ albumin, sigmoidoscopy/colonoscopy with biopsies, white cell scan, BaFT; tests for malabsorption: vitamin B_{12}, folate, vitamin D, calcium

(Rx) 5-aminosalicylic acid (5-ASA) (e.g. mesalazine), steroids, antibiotics, azathioprine/6-mercaptopurine, methotrexate, infliximab (anti TNF-α [tissue necrosis factor-α]), enteral therapies (elemental diet, TPN [total parenteral nutrition]), surgery

(Cx) Stricturing, bowel obstruction, perforation, cholelithiasis, fatty liver

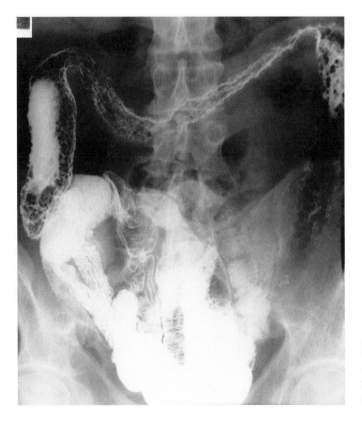

Figure 1.21
Cobblestone mucosa of the colon in Crohn's disease

ULCERATIVE COLITIS

P Involves the rectum and extends proximally; inflammation confined to mucosa and submucosa; distorted crypt architecture, cryptitis, crypt abscesses, inflammatory cell infiltrate, vascular congestion

A Genetic predisposition, non-smokers

Sy Diarrhoea, rectal bleeding and mucus, abdominal pain

Si Weight loss, fever, erythema nodosum, pyoderma gangrenosum

Ix ↑ CRP, ↑ ESR, ↑ platelets, ↓ albumin, ↓ Hb (haemoglobin); stool microscopy/culture, abdominal X-ray (AXR) (need to rule out toxic dilatation), sigmoidoscopy with biopsies, pANCA +ve (~70 per cent)

Rx 5-ASA, steroids, azathioprine/6-mercaptopurine, ciclosporin, surgery

Cx Haemorrhage, toxic megacolon, colorectal carcinoma, fatty liver, primary sclerosing cholangitis

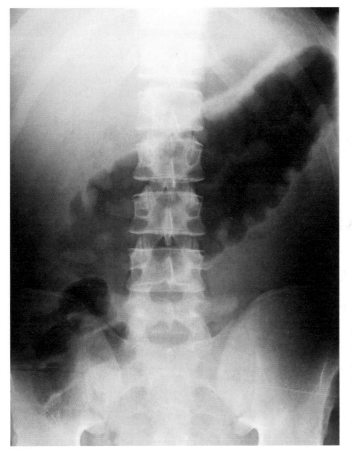

Figure 1.22 Toxic megacolon: dilatation of the transverse colon with loss of the normal haustral pattern and extensive mucosal irregularity

Table 1.2 Differences between Crohn's disease and ulcerative colitis

	Crohn's disease	Ulcerative colitis
Distribution	Can affect any part of GI tract – from mouth to anus	Affects large bowel only
Endoscopy findings	Rectum frequently spared	Rectum always affected
	Some areas of healthy bowel between diseased segments (skip lesions)	Continuous inflammation
	Bowel wall is thickened and has 'cobblestone' appearance due to deep ulceration	Bowel wall is thin and featureless in severe disease
Histology	Granuloma is characteristic finding	Inflammation usually confined to mucosa
	Transmural inflammation (extends all the way through the bowel wall)	
Radiology	Strictures, fissures and fistulae are common	Less common in ulcerative colitis
	Asymmetrical inflammation	Symmetrical inflammation
Smoking	Strongly associated with smoking	Associated with non-smokers or ex-smokers
	Predicts a worse course of disease Increases risk of surgery and further surgery	Appears to protect against disease

INFECTIOUS DIARRHOEA

(P) Organisms causing diarrhoea produce their effect by invasion and destruction of mucosal cells, and toxin production

(A) Travel, contact, age (<5 years and >70 years have increased mortality), food, recent antibiotic use (*Clostridium difficile*)

(S) Fever, diarrhoea (?bloody), nausea, dehydration, abdominal pain
Bloody diarrhoea is more common with *Campylobacter*, *Shigella*

(Ix) FBC, U&E, CRP, stool microscopy, culture and sensitivity (MC&S), blood cultures if septic

(Rx) Majority of cases are self-terminating and require rehydration and electrolyte correction; antibiotics are considered in immunocompromised patients, the very young or the very septic; always liaise with microbiologists

(Cx) Renal failure, septic shock; *E. coli* is associated with the haemolytic–uraemic syndrome

DYSPEPSIA[2]

(P) 'Dyspepsia' encompasses a group of symptoms, including heartburn, nausea, epigastric/retrosternal pain, bloating, anorexia and early satiety. Several disorders can cause dyspepsia, including peptic ulcers, oesophagitis, gastritis, gastric cancer and gallstones.

(S) *Alarm symptoms/signs*: unintentional weight loss, unexplained iron deficiency, dysphagia, GI bleeding, persistent continuous vomiting, epigastric mass, previous gastric surgery, previous gastric ulcer

GASTRO-OESOPHAGEAL REFLUX DISEASE (GORD)

(P) Decreased lower oesophageal sphincter tone; sustained or transient

(A) Usually no obvious cause; secondary causes include smoking, pregnancy, scleroderma, drugs, trauma, alcohol, obesity

Helicobacter pylori is **not** associated with GORD

(Sy) Heartburn, regurgitation

(Ix) OGD, 24-h pH monitoring in difficult cases

(Rx) *Conservative*: weight loss, avoidance of smoking and alcohol

Medical: simple antacids, H_2 blockers (e.g. ranitidine), proton pump inhibitor (PPI) (e.g. omeprazole)

Surgery: Nissen fundoplication (see p. 110)

(Cx) Reflux oesophagitis, peptic stricture, Barrett's oesophagus

BARRETT'S OESOPHAGUS

(P) Squamous → columnar metaplasia in lower oesophagus, premalignant

(A) Secondary to chronic GORD

(S) As GORD

(Ix) Serial OGDs to detect progression of dysplasia

(Rx) Surgical removal, endoscopic ablation

(Cx) Adenocarcinoma

PEPTIC ULCER DISEASE

(P) Break in mucosal surface >5 mm

(A) *Helicobacter pylori* is associated with 95 per cent duodenal ulcers and 70 per cent gastric ulcers; NSAIDs, smoking, alcohol

(S) As above

(Ix) Anyone >55 years with new-onset dyspepsia, or anyone with alarm symptoms should undergo an OGD and testing for *H. pylori*; if <55 years with no alarm symptoms, then the patient can simply undergo a urea breath test, FBC

(Rx) Antacids, H_2-receptor blockers, eradication of *H. pylori*, PPI, sucralfate, avoidance of smoking, NSAIDs and alcohol

All patients with gastric ulcers should have repeat OGD to ensure healing

(Cx) GI bleed, perforation, gastric outlet obstruction

REFERENCES

1   Thomas PD, Forbes A, Green J *et al*. Guidelines for the investigation of chronic diarrhoea, 2nd edition. *Gut* 2003;52(Suppl V):v1–v15.

2   National Institute for Clinical Excellence. *NICE clinical guideline 17: Dyspepsia: management of dyspepsia in adults in primary care*. London: National Institute for Clinical Excellence, 2004.

HEPATOLOGY

HEPATOLOGY INVESTIGATIONS

Blood tests
- **Hepatocellular integrity:**
  - alanine transaminase (ALT)/aspartate transaminase (AST)
  - lactate dehydrogenase (LDH): markedly raised in liver metastases and obstructive jaundice
  - gamma glutamyl transferase (GGT): raised in hepatocellular, hepatobiliary and alcoholic liver disease
  - iron/ferritin: raised in haemochromatosis, liver necrosis, alcoholic liver disease, acute viral hepatitis
- **Disorders of excretion:**
  - bilirubin: jaundice occurs at levels >40 mmol/L:

    > **Hyperbilirubinaemia:**
    > Indirect bilirubin is produced as a water-insoluble, albumin-bound form which is conjugated in the liver to form direct bilirubin, a water-soluble form.
    >   Jaundice can be divided into three forms:
    > 1 pre-hepatic: due to haemolysis – LDH:AST ratio >12, no bilirubinuria
    > 2 intrahepatic: hepatocellular damage – LDH:AST ratio <12, bilirubinuria
    > 3 post-hepatic: due to cholestasis, bilirubinuria

  - alkaline phosphatase (ALP): raised in cholestasis (NB also found in bone, kidney, intestine and lung – isoenzymes can differentiate the source)
  - total copper: raised in cholestasis; decreased in Wilson's disease
  - cholesterol: marked increase in cholestasis
- **Synthetic function:**
  - coagulation: clotting factors I, II, V, VII, XI–XIII are synthesized in the liver; monitored using prothrombin time (PT)/international normalized ratio (INR)
  - albumin
  - A preliminary 'liver screen' includes: viral hepatitis serology, cytomegalovirus (CMV), Epstein–Barr virus (EBV), autoantibodies, immunoglobulin levels, ferritin, copper, caeruloplasmin, α_1-antitrypsin, α-fetoprotein, Ca 19-9, amylase and ultrasonography

Imaging
- **USS:** can comment on echogenicity, nodularity, lesions and the biliary system; Doppler can assess venous flow
- **CT:** gives further details of hepatic parenchyma; contrast media is used in triple phase CT (looking at the arterial, parenchymal and venous phase) to help differentiate between liver parenchyma and pathological structures
- **MRI:** allows cross- and longitudinal sections; further differentiation between tissues than USS and CT; MR angiography and MRCP (cholangiopancreatography) available
- **Angiography:** delineates vascular supply to liver
- **Nuclear medicine**

Liver biopsy
- Can be done directly at the bedside, under ultrasound guidance or via the transjugular (TJ) route. TJ biopsies are less readily available and usually reserved for high-risk patients, in whom bleeding is more likely

CIRRHOSIS

P Necrosis of hepatic parenchyma with connective tissue proliferation and nodular regeneration

A Multiple causes, discussed below; commonest cause is chronic alcohol abuse

Ix Investigations are aimed at finding the cause

LFT, FBC, U&E

Albumin and coagulation to assess synthetic function

Liver biopsy will show degree of activity and fibrosis and help diagnose a cause

S Related to the underlying cause: lethargy, splenomegaly, jaundice, leuconychia, telangiectasia, spider naevi, gynaecomastia, xanthelasma/xanthoma, Dupuytren's contracture, clubbing, dilated chest/abdominal wall veins, scratch marks, fetor hepaticus, palmar erythema

Rx Aimed at the underlying cause and preventing complications; supportive treatment includes laxatives (prevent encephalopathy), vitamin K (correct clotting), nutritional support, antibiotics ± liver transplant

The Child–Pugh scoring shown in Table 1.3 is used to predict the prognosis of cirrhotic patients.

Table 1.3 Child–Pugh scoring system for cirrhotic patients

Indices	1 point	2 points	3 points
Albumin (g/L)	>35	30–35	<30
Bilirubin (µmol/L)	<34	34–51	>51
INR	<1.7	1.7–2.3	>2.3
Ascites	No	Mild–moderate	Severe
Encephalopathy	No	Stages I and II	Stages III and IV

Total score: 5–6, Child–Pugh A; 7–9, Child–Pugh B; 10–15 Child–Pugh C

Box 1.13 COMPLICATIONS OF CIRRHOSIS

MALNUTRITION

1 Catabolism
2 Reduced glycogenolysis and increased gluconeogenesis
3 Hypoglycaemia/impaired glucose tolerance

HEPATIC ENCEPHALOPATHY

A Infection, constipation, drugs/toxins, GI bleed, electrolyte disturbance
Si Affects conscious level, behaviour and intellectual function
Ix Psychometric testing, EEG (electroencephalography), ammonia
Rx Removal of causative factors, antibiotics, laxatives, branched-chain amino acids

ASCITES/OEDEMA

P Portal hypertension, hypoalbuminaemia and increased capillary permeability leads to fluid seepage, with stimulation of the renin–angiotensin system
S Abdominal distension, breathlessness with gross ascites
Ix Ascitic aspirate: protein, cell count, microscopy/culture, cytology
Cx Spontaneous bacterial peritonitis (white cell count [WCC] >250/mm³), respiratory compromise, hernia, compression of renal vein/IVC (inferior vena cava), hepatorenal syndrome, encephalopathy, electrolyte disturbance

- **Rx** Fluid restriction, salt restriction, diuretics, paracentesis, TIPS (transjugular intrahepatic portosystemic shunt, see Information Box, p. 39)

VITAMIN DEFICIENCY

Typically B vitamins (especially thiamine)

COAGULOPATHY

IMPAIRED IMMUNE SYSTEM

VARICES

- **P** Portal hypertension leads to the formation of collateral circulations; occur when portal pressure exceeds 12 mmHg
- **Rx** *Acute variceal bleed*: ABC, fluid resuscitation, endoscopic treatment (sclerosant, band ligation), balloon tamponade (Sengstaken–Blakemore tube), terlipressin, antibiotics
  Prevention: β-blockers (propranolol), endoscopic screening, TIPS, liver transplantation

HEPATORENAL SYNDROME

Renal failure in the presence of severe liver disease, where all other causes have been excluded

HEPATOCELLULAR CARCINOMA (HCC)

Cirrhosis is found in 65–90 per cent of patients with HCC

ALCOHOLISM

- **P** Steatosis, fibrosis, cirrhosis
- **A** Degree of liver damage dependent on genetic susceptibility and coexisting liver disease; women progress to cirrhosis faster
- **S** CAGE questionnaire:
  - do you feel you should Cut down your alcohol consumption?
  - do you feel Annoyed when people criticize your drinking?
  - do you feel Guilty?
  - do you ever drink first thing in the morning – an Eye-opener?

  Otherwise, the symptoms/signs depend on the degree of liver damage
- **Ix** As for cirrhosis: LFT (↑GGT), ↓albumin, coagulation, FBC: ↑MCV (mean corpuscular volume), ↓platelets, U&E, ↑IgA, ↑cholesterol; USS; liver biopsy will give the exact degree of damage, but is not required for diagnosis
- **Rx** Abstinence, nutrition, vitamin replacement, laxatives, liver transplantation

ACUTE ALCOHOLIC HEPATITIS

- **S** Fever, nausea, RUQ (right upper quadrant) pain, jaundice, ascites, oedema, encephalopathy
- **Rx** All the above measures ± steroids/pentoxifylline
- **Px** Mortality rate ~10 per cent

HEPATIC FAILURE

There are three types of acute liver failure:

1. *hyperacute or fulminant liver failure* – encephalopathy develops within 1 week

2.   *acute liver failure* – encephalopathy develops within 2–4 weeks

3.   *subacute liver failure* – encephalopathy develops within 4–8 weeks.

P   Acute necrotizing hepatitis leading to cell destruction

A   Viral hepatitis, infections (viral, bacterial, parasitic), drugs, toxins, alcohol, ischaemic, complications associated with pregnancy, malignancy

Sy   Lethargy, weakness, nausea, anorexia, sleep disturbance

Si   Jaundice, fever, fetor hepaticus, encephalopathy, cerebral oedema leading to bradycardia, hypertension, tachypnoea

Ix   Liver screen to look for an underlying cause; poor prognostic indicators include: ↑bilirubin, severe hyponatraemia, rising lactate, acidosis, rapid drop in transaminases, renal failure

Cx   Renal failure, coagulopathy, respiratory failure, sepsis, circulatory failure, hypoglycaemia, pancreatitis

Rx   Supportive treatment in an intensive care setting; liver transplantation

BUDD–CHIARI SYNDROME

P   Hepatic venous outflow obstruction; this leads to increased hepatic sinusoidal pressure and portal hypertension

A   Hypercoagulable states; myeloproliferative disorders are the most common cause

S   Depends on speed of onset; abdominal pain, hepatomegaly, ascites; varices and splenomegaly can be seen in the chronic form; nausea and jaundice in the acute form

Ix   ↑↑ALT/AST, ↑ALP/bilirubin, ↓albumin, USS with Doppler studies of the hepatic vein, CT/MRI

Rx   Anticoagulation

Ascites is controlled with sodium restriction and diuretics ± paracentesis

Thrombolysis, angioplasty, TIPS, liver transplant

INFORMATION BOX: TIPS

A **T**ransjugular **I**ntrahepatic **P**ortosystemic **S**hunt is a procedure performed by a radiologist whereby a connection is made between the portal vein and the hepatic vein via a catheter introduced into the jugular vein. This aims to reduce the portal hypertension causing some of the symptoms of liver disease, but can precipitate encephalopathy.

VIRAL HEPATITIS

HEPATITIS A VIRUS (HAV)

P   RNA virus; transmitted by faecal-oral route. Does not cause cirrhosis

A   Poor hygiene correlates with increased risk

Sy   Nausea, anorexia, vomiting, diarrhoea, weakness, fever, malaise, arthralgia, dark urine

Si   Jaundice, hepatomegaly, splenomegaly, lymphadenopathy

Ix   LFT: raised transaminases and bilirubin, HAV IgM (immunoglobulin M)

Rx   Supportive

HEPATITIS B VIRUS (HBV)

P DNA virus

A Parenteral, sexual, vertical transmission

Sy Similar to hepatitis A, but often more severe; often found on antenatal testing

Si Jaundice, pruritus, tender hepatomegaly, lymphadenopathy, splenomegaly

Ix See Box 1.14

Box 1.14 SEROLOGY IN HEPATITIS B INFECTION

- *HBsAg*: first serological marker; usually becomes undetectable at 6 months
- *HBsAb*: detectable once HBsAg clears; remains indefinitely
- *HBcAg*: not detected routinely
- *HBcAb*: detectable 1–2 weeks after HBsAg (IgM initially, then IgG)
- *HBeAg*: occurs shortly after HBsAg; correlates with viral replication
- *HBeAb*: correlates with lower viral replication and infectivity
- *HBV DNA by PCR* (polymerase chain reaction): quantifies viral replication

HBsAg, hepatitis B surface antigen; HBsAb, hepatitis B surface antibody; HBcAg, hepatitis B core antigen; HBcAb, hepatitis B core antibody; HBeAg, hepatitis B e antigen, HBeAb, hepatitis B e antibody

---

Rx alcohol avoidance, antivirals e.g. lamivudine, interferon alfa

Cx >90 per cent patients will clear the virus

Carrier state: HBsAg persists for >6 months with no signs of acute hepatitis

10–20 per cent of carriers will develop cirrhosis

↑ risk of hepatocellular carcinoma

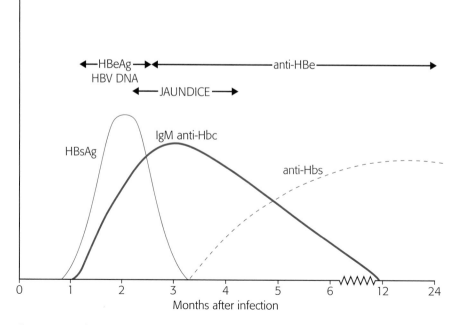

Figure 1.23 Changes in hepatitis B enzymes after acute infection

HEPATITIS C VIRUS (HCV)

- **(P)** RNA virus; six genotypes
- **(A)** Spread parenterally or sporadically
- **(Sy)** Prodromal symptoms usually mild or absent; fatigue may be pronounced
- **(Si)** Jaundice, hepatomegaly
- **(Ix)** HCV antibody, HCV RNA by PCR
- **(Rx)** Antiviral therapy: usually peginterferon alfa and ribavirin, although many new treatments in development
- **(Cx)** >80 per cent develop chronic HCV infection

    ~30 per cent develop cirrhosis

    ↑ risk of hepatocellular carcinoma

HEPATITIS D VIRUS (HDV)

- **(P)** RNA virus, dependent on presence of HBV for infectivity
- **(A)** Corresponds to HBV infection
- **(S)** As for HBV
- **(Ix)** HDAg, HDV RNA by PCR

    Anti-HDV and RNA are markers of replication; persistent HDV antibody is consistent with chronic HDV
- **(Rx)** Treatment is usually supportive; limited response to antivirals

    Prevention is only by immunity to HBV; HBV carriers should avoid HDV endemic areas
- **(Cx)** As for HBV

HEPATITIS E VIRUS (HEV)

- **(P)** RNA virus, faecal–oral transmission
- **(S)** Very similar to hepatitis A
- **(Ix)** HEV antibody, HEV RNA
- **(Rx)** Supportive, prevention by improvements in sanitation
- **(Cx)** Fulminant hepatic failure: 20 per cent incidence in pregnant women

AUTOIMMUNE DISEASE

AUTOIMMUNE HEPATITIS (AIH)

- **(P)** Periportal piecemeal necrosis/bridging necrosis; fibrosis
- **(A)** More common in young women
- **(Sy)** Fatigue, abdominal discomfort, decreased appetite, myalgia
- **(Si)** Hepatomegaly, icterus, signs of chronic liver disease/cirrhosis
- **(Ix)** Raised transaminases, ↑ ESR, ANA +ve, smooth muscle antibody +ve, anti-LKM (liver, kidney, microsomal antibodies) +ve, ↑ IgG, liver biopsy
- **(Rx)** Steroids, azathioprine, ursodeoxycholic acid (UDCA), liver transplantation

PRIMARY BILIARY CIRRHOSIS (PBC)

- **(P)** Chronic inflammation and destruction of the small and medium bile ducts
- **(A)** 80–90 per cent women; age 30–60 years

(S) Fatigue, pruritus, arthralgia, xanthelasma, hepatomegaly, splenomegaly, jaundice, signs of chronic liver disease, osteoporosis

(Ix) cholestatic LFTs; ↑IgM, antimitochondrial antibody (AMA) +ve (in ~95 per cent), ANA +ve (in ~40 per cent), liver biopsy

(Rx) *Pruritus*: colestyramine, UDCA, antihistamines
Osteoporosis and hypercholesterolaemia: bisphosphonates, statins
Immunosuppression: prednisolone, azathioprine
Liver transplantation

PRIMARY SCLEROSING CHOLANGITIS (PSC)

(P) Progressive fibrosis and obliteration of the biliary ducts

(A) 70 per cent men; 3rd–5th decade; associated with inflammatory bowel disease (mainly ulcerative colitis)

(S) Can be asymptomatic; fatigue, weight loss, fever, pruritus, RUQ discomfort, hepatomegaly; may have relapsing cholangitis

(Ix) Cholestatic LFTs; pANCA +ve, ANA +ve, ↑IgM, MRCP/ERCP (endoscopic retrograde cholangiopancreatography), liver biopsy

(Rx) *Medical*: UDCA, prednisolone and methotrexate
Endoscopy: therapeutic ERCP: sphincterotomy/stent insertion
Surgery: liver transplantation

METABOLIC DISORDERS

NON-ALCOHOLIC STEATOHEPATITIS (NASH)

(P) When liver fat content >12 per cent = fatty liver; this can lead to inflammation and fibrosis

(A) ♀ > ♂
Viral hepatitis and autoimmune conditions **must** be excluded
Multiple other causes – commonest are obesity, diabetes and hyperlipidaemia

(S) Often asymptomatic and found after routine blood tests reveal abnormal LFTs, hepatomegaly, fatigue

(Ix) LFT-raised transaminases, liver screen to rule out other causes of liver disease, lipid screen, HbA_{1c}, USS, liver biopsy is diagnostic

(Rx) No specific treatments; aim at removing any causative factors; alcohol abstinence

HEREDITARY HAEMOCHROMATOSIS (HHC)

(P) Autosomal recessive mutations in the *HFE* gene leading to abnormal absorption of iron

(A) ♂:♀ ratio = 5–10:1

(Si) Iron overload in multiple sites throughout the body, leading to a wide variety of signs: hepatomegaly, stigmata of chronic liver disease, ascites, splenomegaly, fatigue, arthralgia, pigmentation

(Sy) Symptoms of cardiomyopathy, diabetes mellitus, hypothyroidism, hypogonadism, hypoparathyroidism

(Ix) ↑ferritin, iron and transferrin saturation; HFE genotyping and family genotyping; raised transaminases, ↑IgG, USS/CT/MRI, liver biopsy

Venesection, desferrioxamine, low iron diet, alcohol abstinence, liver transplantation, screening for HCC

 HCC, liver failure

WILSON'S DISEASE

P Autosomal recessive; abnormal hepatobiliary copper excretion

S Related to the degree and sites of copper deposition

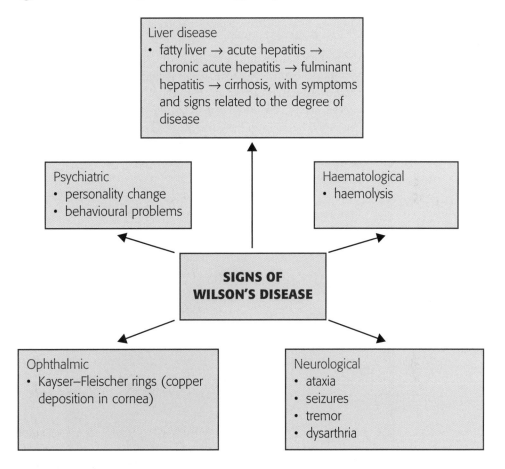

Figure 1.24 Signs of Wilson's disease

Ix ↑ serum free copper and urinary copper, ↓ caeruloplasmin, USS, liver biopsy, penicillamine test
To assess other organ involvement: slit lamp eye examination, MRI, ECG, echo, EEG, EMG (electromyogram)

Rx D-penicillamine (chelates copper), low copper diet, liver transplantation

INFECTIONS

LIVER ABSCESS

 Bacterial, helminthic, fungal or protozoal
Spread via blood, post-traumatic, directly or via the biliary tree

Fever, RUQ pain/tenderness, right-sided pleural effusion, septicaemia, rupture

FBC, LFT, CRP, ESR, CXR, USS ± CT, angiography is required to assess arterial anatomy pre-operatively, USS/CT-guided aspiration

Intravenous antibiotics, aspiration, percutaneous drainage, surgery

HYDATID DISEASE

Majority due to *Echinococcus cysticus*, a tapeworm; commonly found in areas of cattle breeding; spread via faecal–oral route
Larvae travel to the portal system via the intestine and form fluid-filled cysts (hydatids) in the liver; these can grow up to 1 cm/year

RUQ pain once the cyst is large enough

Hepatomegaly due to hydatid growth

Eosinophilia, LFT, serology, USS

~10 per cent spontaneously regress; surgical removal, mebendazole/albendazole

Rupture of the hydatid will cause an anaphylactic reaction

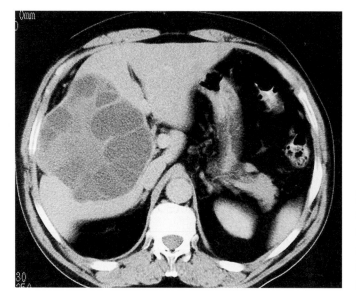

Figure 1.25 Hydatid cyst: a well-delineated multiloculated cystic mass, with orderly internal septations, in the right lobe of the liver

HEPATIC TUMOURS

HEPATIC ADENOMA

Vary in size and number, usually solitary and found in the right lobe

Found in women in their reproductive years; often associated with oral contraceptives

Usually asymptomatic and found by chance; if large they may be associated with abdominal discomfort; haemorrhage: severe pain

LFTs normal; USS, CT, MRI, liver biopsy
 Embolization, surgery

HEPATOCELLULAR CARCINOMA (HCC)

A Affects all age groups; slight increased incidence in men (ratio 2–3:1)
Liver disease: cirrhosis, HBV, HCV, HDV, haemochromatosis, α_1-antitrypsin deficiency, autoimmune hepatitis, PBC
Alcohol, smoking; drugs, genetics

Sy Weight loss, anorexia, abdominal pain

Si Cachexia, hepatomegaly, fever, lymphadenopathy
Metastases may also add to the symptoms and signs: lungs, bone, lymph nodes

Ix Raised transaminases, ↑ alpha-fetoprotein, CRP and ESR may be raised; there may be cholestasis if the tumour affects the intrahepatic bile ducts; USS (microbubble contrast), CT, MRI; liver biopsy (only if diagnosis is in question, as the procedure may cause tumour spread)

Rx Resection, liver transplant, chemoembolization, ethanol injection, laser ablation

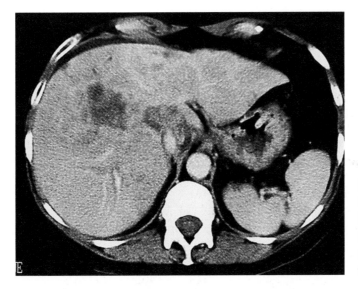

Figure 1.26
Hepatocellular carcinoma: localized poorly marginated mixed density area in the right lobe of the liver

NEUROLOGY

NEUROLOGY INVESTIGATIONS

- **CT:** study of choice in acute trauma and haemorrhage; usually given with contrast to help enhance tumours, infections and infarcts
- **MRI:** T_1-weighted images enhance acute haemorrhage; T_2-weighted images enhance oedema, infarction, demyelination and chronic haemorrhage
- **Angiography** can also be performed with or without contrast
- **EEG:** electrodes are places on the scalp and electrical activity of the brain is recorded; particularly important in evaluating epilepsy
- **Evoked potentials:** electrical potentials are measured while nerves are repetitively stimulated; the commonest use is in visual evoked potentials to diagnose multiple sclerosis
- **Nerve conduction studies:** nerves are stimulated and the electrical activity is measured from different points; conduction velocity can be recorded
- **EMG:** electromyography records electrical potentials from needle electrodes in muscle at rest and during contraction; this can differentiate between neuropathic and myopathic disorders
- **Lumbar puncture:** cerebrospinal fluid (CSF) is taken via a needle inserted into the spinal column between L3/4 or L4/5
- **Tensilon test:** a short-acting anticholinesterase (edrophonium) is given intravenously to see if there is any improvement in those with suspected myasthenia gravis

ISCHAEMIA

CEREBROVASCULAR DISEASE/ISCHAEMIC STROKE

(P) Acute occlusion of an intracranial vessel leading to hypoxia and infarction; if blood flow is restored prior to significant cell death there may be transient symptoms: **transient ischaemic attack (TIA)**

(A) Diabetes mellitus, hypertension, smoking, hypercholesterolaemia, family history, age, atrial fibrillation, valvular lesions, cardiac congenital defects, hypercoagulable states, vasculitis

(S) Symptoms are always variable and dependent on the exact area and arteries involved; Box 1.15 gives an idea of symptoms related to territories.

Box 1.15 SYMPTOMS OF CEREBROVASCULAR DISEASE ACCORDING TO TERRITORIES

Anterior cerebral artery occlusion
- Contralateral hemiplegia
- Gait apraxia
- Abulia (severe apathy)
- Urinary incontinence
- Lower limb sensory loss

Middle cerebral artery occlusion
- Contralateral hemiplegia
- Homonymous hemianopia
- Contralateral sensory loss

- Dysarthria, dysphasia
  Non-dominant symptoms include:
  - Aphasia
  - Neglect
  - Constructional apraxia

Posterior cerebral artery occlusion
- Homonymous hemianopia ± macular sparing
- Contralateral hemiplegia
- Ataxia/hemiballismus
- Visual agnosia
- Cortical blindness

Posterior inferior cerebellar artery (PICA) occlusion
- Syncope
- Vertigo
- Hemiplegia
- Dysarthria
- Ipsilateral face numbness
- Contralateral limb numbness

Basilar artery occlusion
- Dizziness
- Vertigo
- Diplopia
- Dysarthria
- Facial numbness
- Ipsilateral hemiparesis

 CT, MRI, MR angiography, carotid dopplers, echo, ECG

 Medical: aspirin, clopidogrel, dipyridamole, anticoagulation
Thrombolysis is not yet in widespread use
Collateral blood flow is blood pressure dependent, therefore BP should not be lowered unless there are signs of malignant hypertension
Surgery: carotid endarterectomy

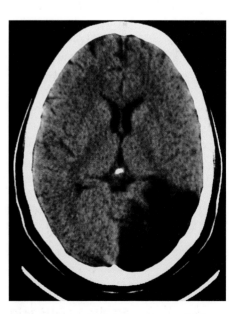

Figure 1.27 Large left posterior cerebral artery infarct

CEREBELLAR SYNDROME

A Vascular lesion, alcohol, demyelination, tumours, paraneoplastic phenomenon, hypothyroidism, phenytoin toxicity, metabolic disorders (e.g. Wilson's disease)

Sy Poor balance, dysphasia

Si 'DANISH', see Box 1.16

Box 1.16 FEATURES OF CEREBELLAR SYNDROMES

Dysdiadochokinesis
Ataxia
Nystagmus
Intention tremor, past pointing
Scanning speech, dysarthria
Hypotonia, hyporeflexia

Ix MRI

Rx Treatment aimed at underlying disorder

INFECTION

MENINGITIS

P Infection of the meninges; commonest pathogen is *Streptococcus pneumoniae*; other bacterial pathogens include *Neisseria meningitidis*, *Haemophilus influenzae*, *Listeria monocytogenes* and *Mycobacterium tuberculosis*
Can also be caused by viruses and fungal infection

A Higher risk in immunosuppressed individuals

Sy Headache, photophobia, nausea, vomiting, neck pain

Si Fever, neck stiffness, confusion, drowsiness, petechiae, Kernig's sign (hamstring spasm when attempting to straighten leg)

Ix FBC, U&E, LFT, coagulation, blood cultures, CXR, lumbar puncture (LP). NB do **not** perform LP if patient has a petechial rash, without the results of clotting profile (need to exclude DIC [disseminated intravascular coagulation]); if there are any neurological signs or conscious level is reduced, perform a CT head prior to LP (? brain abscess)
CSF samples can also be sent for PCR to identify meningococcus, AFB and viruses

Table 1.4 Lumbar puncture results

	Neutrophils (×10⁶/L)	Lymphocytes (×10⁶/L)	Protein (g/L)	Glucose (ratio CSF/ serum)
Normal	0	<5	<0.4	>0.6
Bacterial	↑↑↑	↑	>1.0	<0.4
Viral	↑	↑↑↑	0.4–1.0	Usually normal
Tuberculosis	↑	↑↑↑	>1.0	<0.4

Rx Start empirical antibiotics immediately; most hospitals advocate third generation cephalosporins (e.g. cefotaxime), plus ampicillin if *Listeria* is suspected
Specific treatment for TB can usually be held off until CSF results are available

Chemoprophlaxis is often offered to close contacts of meningococcal meningitis (e.g. rifampicin)

Close liaison with microbiologist is essential

Cx Seizures, hydrocephalus, cerebral venous/sagittal sinus thrombosis, neurological sequelae, DIC, multi-organ failure, death

ENCEPHALITIS

P Infection of the brain parenchyma

A Can be primary or secondary to viral infections from other areas of the body; 10 per cent caused by herpes simplex virus, which is dealt with here

S Prodromal viral symptoms; headaches, fever, meningism, confusion, delirium, seizures, neurological deficits

Ix FBC, U&E, clotting, septic screen

Specific tests: MRI, EEG, LP with CSF results as for viral meningitis, CSF HSV PCR

Rx Aciclovir; supportive and symptomatic treatment (e.g. for seizures) with close liaison with microbiologist and ITU

Cx Fatal if untreated and causes death in 7–10 days; neurological sequelae e.g. seizures, amnesia, motor deficits etc.

DEMYELINATION

MULTIPLE SCLEROSIS (MS)

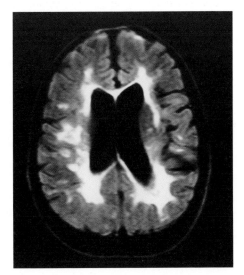

Figure 1.28 Multiple areas of increased signal in the periventricular deep white matter are demyelination plaques in multiple sclerosis

P Chronic disease of the central nervous system (CNS), characterized by white plaques (areas of demyelination and perivascular inflammation) occurring anywhere within the CNS

A Affects people within their reproductive years; ? immune dysfunction ? viral association

Incidence ↑ with distance from the equator

S Symptoms depend on the position of plaques; usually follows a relapsing–remitting course

Commoner presentations include internuclear ophthalmoplegia (see Fig. 1.29), optic neuritis, cerebellar syndrome, weakness, sensory disturbance, Lhermitte's sign (electric sensation down spine on neck flexion)

Ix Lumbar puncture/CSF (↑ protein, ↑ immunoglobulin levels, oligoclonal bands), visual evoked potentials, MRI (demyelinating lesions)

Rx High-dose steroids for exacerbations; interferon-β; treatments for muscle spasm (e.g. baclofen), tremor (e.g. clonazepam), pain (e.g. gabapentin), urinary incontinence (e.g. anticholinergics), antidepressants

Px Increased risk of suicide; mean prognosis 25–35 years

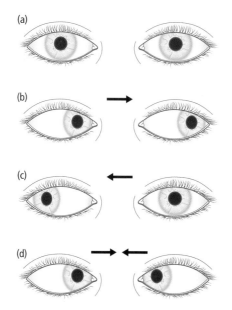

Figure 1.29 Left internuclear ophthalmoplegia. The lesion affects the left medial longitudinal fasciculus (MLF) and prevents adduction of the ipsilateral eye during conjugate gaze (c); convergence is usually normal (d)

GUILLAIN–BARRÉ SYNDROME

P Autoimmune response causing demyelination

A Usually follows a respiratory or GI infection; associated with infections, malignancies, drugs, pregnancy, vaccinations

Sy Progressive ascending weakness, sensory loss, paraesthesia, pain, dysphasia, dysarthria

Si Dysreflexia, hypotonia, papilloedema, bulbar palsy, labile vital signs due to autonomic involvement

Cranial nerves are involved in 45–70 per cent

Ix Pregnancy test, LFT (↑), lumbar puncture (↑ CSF protein; normal cell counts), nerve conduction studies (may take 2–3 weeks to develop abnormalities), antibody screen, ECG, MRI, spirometry

Rx Intravenous immunoglobulin, plasmapheresis; close monitoring for cardiac arrhythmias and respiratory failure, and close liaison with ITU; DVT (deep vein thrombosis) prophylaxis

Cx Mortality 5–10 per cent; autonomic lability, pneumonia, respiratory failure, cardiac arrhythmias, neurological sequelae

AUTOIMMUNE DISORDERS

MYASTHENIA GRAVIS

 Autoimmune condition with antibodies directed against the acetylcholine receptors on the post-synaptic muscle membrane

Thymus is abnormal in ~75 per cent: 65 per cent have hyperplastic thymus, ~10 per cent have thymic tumours; prevalence 1 in 7500; ♀:♂ 3:2

Weakness and fatiguability; often affects cranial muscles early leading to ptosis, diplopia, dysarthria, dysphagia; limb weakness is often proximal
If respiratory function is affected this is a myasthenic crisis

Acetylcholine receptor antibodies, CXR/CT (to look at the thymus), anticholinesterase/edrophonium test (Tensilon test), nerve conduction studies, thyroid function, spirometry

Medical: anticholinesterases e.g. pyridostigmine
Surgery: thymectomy: improvement in ~85 per cent of patients
Immunosuppression: steroids, azathioprine, ciclosporin, mycophenolate mofetil, cyclophosphamide (rarely)
Emergency treatment: intravenous immunoglobulins, plasmapheresis

PERIPHERAL NEUROPATHY

 Sensory neuropathy: diabetes, alcohol, rheumatoid arthritis, drugs, malignancy, B$_{12}$ deficiency, chronic renal failure
Motor neuropathy: Guillain–Barré syndrome, lead toxicity, porphyria, Charcot–Marie–Tooth disease

Commonly there is a sensory loss in a stocking distribution; usually a full history and examination will give clues as to the underlying cause

 Urine dipstick, blood sugar, FBC, B$_{12}$ levels, history of alcohol consumption

Aimed at underlying cause

CHARCOT–MARIE–TOOTH DISEASE/HEREDITARY MOTOR AND SENSORY NEUROPATHY (HMSN)

 Several types of hereditary motor and sensory neuropathies, classified according to the genetic mutations
Neuronal degeneration; caused by mutations to genes coding the proteins involved in the structure or function of nerve axons or myelin sheaths

 Inherited disorder; mostly autosomal dominant, but there are X-linked varieties

Gradual onset; some asymptomatic patients are picked up on screening
Loss of balance, foot deformities (high arches/hammer toes), weakness

Weakness, atrophy, hyporeflexia/areflexia, sensory loss, nerve enlargement

NCS (nerve conduction studies), EMG, nerve biopsy, genetic testing
Differential diagnosis: need to exclude other causes of neuropathy, including infectious, immunological, endocrinological causes, and vitamin and nutritional deficiencies

 Physiotherapy, occupational therapy, orthopaedic devices to maintain mobility, analgesia

Normal life expectancy

NERVE DISORDERS

FACIAL NERVE PALSY

 Bell's palsy, acoustic neuromas, multiple sclerosis, infarcts, tumours, Lyme disease, sarcoidosis
Ramsay Hunt syndrome: facial palsy due to herpes zoster affecting the geniculate ganglion

S Facial weakness
Upper motor neurone palsy: the frontalis and orbicularis oculi function are preserved i.e. the patient can raise their eyebrows
Lower motor neurone palsy: this function is lost
Ramsay Hunt syndrome: vesicular eruptions of herpes zoster
Acoustic neuromas: involvement of the 8th cranial nerve
Sarcoidosis: parotid gland enlargement/tenderness

Ix Bell's palsy/Ramsay Hunt syndrome (lower motor neurone palsy) do not require further investigation; other conditions listed are described in their own relevant sections

Rx *Medical*: steroids for Bell's palsy, aciclovir if any evidence of herpes zoster
Supportive: taping down eyelids overnight to prevent corneal drying

TRIGEMINAL NEURALGIA

P Pathophysiology unknown ? vascular compression leading to demyelination

A Usually idiopathic; can occur secondary to brain tumours, MS, cranial neuropathies or cerebral aneurysms, but this is rare without other neurological features

Sy Sudden, severe, unilateral electric shock-like or stabbing pain typically felt on one side of the jaw or cheek; affects right side > left side
Triggers include talking, chewing, smiling, brushing teeth, touching the face, or swallowing
Attacks recur at varying intervals (up to hundreds per day) and last for days, weeks, or months at a time, and then remit for months or years
Attacks rarely occur during sleep

Si Neurological examination is normal

Ix No specific investigation required as diagnosis is clinical; if any neurological deficits are present trigeminal neuralgia is unlikely and brain imaging should be performed

Rx Anticonvulsants (carbamazepine, gabapentin); neurosurgical treatment may be required if medical treatment fails

PUPILLARY ABNORMALITIES

HORNER'S SYNDROME/PTOSIS

P Interrupted sympathetic innervation to the eye, at any level from a central lesion to the post-ganglionic fibres

 Central lesions: basal meningitis, demyelinating disease, cerebrovascular accident (CVA), basal skull tumours, pituitary tumour, intrapontine haemorrhage, neck trauma, syringomyelia
Preganglionic lesions: Pancoast's tumour, cervical rib, aneurysm/dissection of aorta, trauma/surgical injury, lesions of the middle ear, neuroblastoma

Post-ganglionic lesions: Herpes zoster, migraine, internal carotid dissection
Drugs: e.g. chlorpromazine, levodopa, prochlorperazine, oral contraceptive pill
(OCP), reserpine

(S) Miosis, ptosis, anhidrosis

(Ix) Diagnosis is clinical; further investigations depend on the location of the lesion, but usually include CT/MRI

(Rx) Aimed at underlying cause

HOLMES–ADIE SYNDROME

(P) Normal variant; rarely a result of a lesion in the efferent parasympathetic pathway

(A) Commoner in young women

(S) Holmes–Adie pupil is a large irregular pupil; pupillary constriction to light (direct and consensual) is slow and incomplete, and the pupil remains constricted for an abnormally long time; usually unilateral
When associated with absent deep tendon jerks, termed Holmes–Adie syndrome

(Ix) Diagnosis is clinical

(Rx) No treatment required

ARGYLL ROBERTSON PUPIL

(A) Neurosyphilis, diabetes mellitus, multiple sclerosis, syringobulbia

(S) Miosis, irregular pupil, absent light reflex, intact accommodation reflex

(Ix) Syphilis serology, urine dipstick (blood/ketones), blood sugar ± CT/MRI brain

(Rx) Based on underlying cause

DEGENERATIVE DISORDERS

ALZHEIMER'S DISEASE (AD)

(P) Cerebral atrophy; neurofibrillary tangles and senile plaques

(A) Most common cause of dementia
Affects >40 per cent of over 80 year olds; <10 per cent are familial

(Sy) Progressive memory loss

(Si) Cognitive impairment; as disease progresses it can affect behaviour, extrapyramidal and cerebellar systems

(Ix) Required to exclude other causes of confusion/memory impairment; this includes FBC, B_{12}, U&E, LFT, TFT, syphilis serology, cortisol, glucose, CT brain; EEG and LP occasionally required to rule out other conditions e.g. Creutzfeldt–Jakob disease (CJD), neurosyphilis, normal pressure hydrocephalus

(Rx) Symptomatic therapy: anxiolytics, antidepressants, antipsychotics; cholinesterase inhibitors (e.g. donepezil), *N*-methyl-D-aspartate antagonists (e.g. memantine)

FRIEDREICH'S ATAXIA

(P) Degeneration of neurones in the spinal column, due to a gene mutation, causing reduction in the protein 'frataxin'; it affects the posterior columns, corticospinal columns, and ventral and lateral spinocerebellar tracts; also affects myocardial and spinal muscle fibres

(A) Autosomal recessive

(S) Onset usually <20 years; foot deformities (hammer toes, clubfoot), ataxia (sensory ± cerebellar), weakness, distal wasting, loss of lower limb tendon reflexes, extensor plantar reflex, gradual sensory loss, nystagmus, dysarthria, dysphagia

(Ix) Genetic testing, MRI (cervical spinal cord atrophy, with no signs of cerebellar atrophy), sensory nerve action potentials (absent in >90 per cent), visual evoked potential (reduced amplitude and delayed), echo, ECG

(Rx) No effective cure or treatment

(Cx) Prognosis 15–20 years; other complications: optic atrophy, deafness, diabetes mellitus, cardiomyopathy, heart block, myocardial fibrosis, scoliosis

PARKINSON'S DISEASE (PD)

(P) Degeneration of the dopaminergic neurones of the substantia nigra

(A) Increased incidence in males, rural living, exposure to well water, positive family history

Important to check drug history to ensure the patient does not have drug-induced parkinsonism (commonly from neuroleptics)

(S) Resting tremor, rigidity, bradykinesia

Other symptoms: masked facies, stooped posture, micrographia, hypophonia, shuffling gait, instability, anosmia, depression, aching pain, sleep disorders, cognitive impairment

(Ix) PD is normally diagnosed clinically

In young (<40 years) patients Wilson's disease (see Hepatology section p. 43) and mass lesions should be ruled out

(Rx) *Medical*: dopamine agonists (cabergoline), levodopa/carbidopa, monoamine oxidase B inhibitor (selegiline), catechol *O*-methyltransferase (COMT) inhibitors (entacapone), anticholinergics, amantadine

Surgery: pallidotomy/thalamotomy (radio-frequency ablation), deep brain stimulation (implanted electrodes)

HUNTINGDON'S DISEASE (HD)

(P) Autosomal dominant; gene on chromosome 4 encodes a protein called *huntingtin*, which accumulates in the brain cells causing damage

(A) Affects males and females equally; usually presents >35 years

(Sy) Involuntary movements, erratic/argumentative behaviour, depression

(Si) Chorea, rigidity, dystonia, loss of saccadic eye movements, behavioural problems, dementia, weight loss

(Ix) Family history is the most important diagnostic tool; DNA analysis to identify the *HD* gene; CT/MRI

(Rx) Nil specific; antidepressants ± tranquillizers to control chorea

(Px) Progressive illness, with death within 15–20 years of diagnosis

MUSCLE DISEASE

MOTOR NEURONE DISEASE (AMYOTROPHIC LATERAL SCLEROSIS)

(P) Degeneration of upper and lower motor neurones, of unknown cause

(A) 5–10 per cent of cases follow an autosomal dominant pattern; the rest are sporadic

♂ > ♀; 40–60 years

S   See Box 1.17

Box 1.17 COMMON PRESENTATIONS OF MOTOR NEURONE DISEASE

- *Spinal muscular atrophy*: limb weakness due to involvement of spinal cord anterior horn cells
- *Primary lateral sclerosis*: spastic limb weakness due to upper motor neurone involvement of the spinal cord
- *Progressive bulbar palsy*: involvement of bulbar motor neurons; it is a progressive disease
- *Amyotrophic lateral sclerosis* (ALS): a mixture of all the above

---

Cardiac and smooth muscle are not involved; ocular muscles very rarely Autonomic dysfunction occurs late; emotional lability (associated with pseudobulbar palsy)

Ix   No specific test; diagnosed clinically when other causes of motor neurone damage have been excluded; EMG confirms fasciculations and fibrillations

Rx   Antispasmodics (e.g. baclofen), glutamate antagonists (e.g. riluzole); emotional and symptomatic support

Cx   Fatal within 3–5 years; death commonly from cardiac arrhythmias or respiratory failure

MYOTONIC DYSTROPHY (DYSTROPHIA MYOTONICA)

P   Autosomal dominant condition
S   Atrophy of temporalis, masseter and facial and neck muscles; dysarthria and dysphagia (secondary to pharyngeal, palatal and tongue involvement), myotonia, frontal balding, mitral valve prolapse, heart block, congestive heart failure, cataracts, intellectual impairment, insulin resistance, hypersomnia
Ix   Diagnosis usually clinical with family history
Creatine kinase (CK), muscle biopsy (showing atrophy), EMG (myotonia)
Rx   Rarely requires treatment; phenytoin very occasionally used

METABOLIC DISORDERS

SUBACUTE COMBINED DEGENERATION OF THE CORD

P B_{12} deficiency leading to degeneration of the posterior column and corticospinal tracts of the spinal cord
A   Pernicious anaemia, dietary deficiency, malabsorption
Sy   Constant and progressive; paraesthesiae, weakness, sensory deficits
Si   Sensorimotor neuropathy, lower limb spasticity, ataxia, extensor plantar response, loss of ankle jerk, optic atrophy/neuritis, variable mood changes
Ix   FBC, B_{12} levels, intrinsic factor antibody
Rx B_{12} replacement
Cx   Prognosis in terms of neurological sequelae is reduced by speed of treatment

MISCELLANEOUS

EPILEPSY

P Abnormal neuronal activity leads to seizures

A Idiopathic, genetic defects, metabolic abnormalities (e.g. alcohol withdrawal, low blood glucose), post-trauma, hypoxic damage, brain tumour, cerebrovascular disease, Alzheimer's disease

---

Box 1.18 CLASSIFICATION OF EPILEPSY

- *Partial seizures*: abnormal electrical discharge originates from discrete regions of the brain; they can be simple (patient fully conscious) or complex (decreased awareness)
- *Generalized seizures*: abnormal electrical discharge involves the entire brain
- *Absence seizures*: 'petit mal'; sudden brief lapses of consciousness without loss of postural control
- *Tonic–clonic seizures*: 'grand mal'; involve jerking movements
- *Atonic seizures*: sudden loss of postural muscle tone; lasts 1–2 s
- *Myoclonic seizures*: sudden contractions of the limbs, usually followed by unconsciousness

---

Ix FBC, U&E, calcium, glucose, magnesium, LFT, urine/serum toxins, EEG, CT/MRI brain, EEG

Rx Anti-epileptics

Cx Status epilepticus

SYRINGOMYELIA/SYRINGOBULBIA

P Formation of a fluid-filled cavity (or syrinx) within the spinal column; when this involves the brainstem it is termed syringobulbia

A Meningeal carcinomatosis, Arnold–Chiari malformation, intramedullary tumours, spinal cord injury, haemorrhage, meningitis, idiopathic

♂ > ♀

S Usually slowly progressive
- Dissociated sensory loss: loss of pain and temperature, while light touch, vibration, and position senses are preserved; it may affect the upper limbs in a 'shawl' distribution
- Muscle atrophy due to extension into the anterior horns of the spinal cord; this begins in the hands and progresses proximally
- Pain
- Lower limb upper motor neurone signs: spasticity, weakness, hyperreflexia
- Autonomic dysfunction

Syringobulbia: characterized by nystagmus, dysphagia, tongue atrophy, palatal weakness and sensory loss in the distribution of the trigeminal nerve

Other manifestations: Charcot joints

Ix MRI; CSF pressure/protein may be raised

Rx Surgery, physiotherapy

NEUROFIBROMATOSIS

 Genetic disorders that affect growth of nerve cells and lead to the formation of tumours on nerves; separated into Type I and Type II

A Autosomal dominant, although many new presentations are due to genetic mutations

S See Box 1.19

Box 1.19 DIAGNOSIS OF NEUROFIBROMATOSIS

Neurofibromatosis 1
Two or more of the following:
Five or more light *café au lait* macules (diameter > 5 mm in prepubertal patients or >15 mm across in postpubertal individuals)
Two or more neurofibromas or one plexiform neurofibroma
First-degree relative with neurofibromatosis 1
Two or more Lisch nodules (iris hamartomas)
Freckling in the armpit or groin areas
Optic glioma
Severe scoliosis
Other bony enlargement or deformity

Neurofibromatosis 2
Bilateral tumours of the VIIIth cranial nerve

or

First-degree relative with neurofibromatosis 2 *plus* unilateral VIIIth cranial nerve tumour

or

Two neurofibroma, glioma, schwannoma, meningioma, or juvenile cataracts

---

Ix Family history, genetic testing, MRI, slit lamp testing for Lisch nodules
Rx Supportive e.g. excision of tumours causing hearing loss or bony deformities
Cx Increased risk of malignancy

MIGRAINE

 Exact pathogenesis unknown; ? vasoconstriction, ? neurotransmitters, ? vasoactive substances

A ♀ > ♂ (ratio 2–3:1)

Sy Headache: throbbing, usually unilateral initially, becoming diffuse over 1–2 h, lasting up to 24 h; nausea/vomiting, photophobia, some have a preceding aura

Si Patients normally have a normal neurological examination; occasional sensory or motor deficits; visual deficits e.g. scotoma, field defects

 Migraines can be diagnosed clinically, but if a patient presents to the emergency department for the first time (especially with neurological deficits) other causes must be excluded

Rx *Prophylaxis*: anti-epileptics, β-blockers, amitriptyline, selective serotonin reuptake inhibitor (SSRI) antidepressants, serotonin antagonists (e.g. methysergide)
Acute attacks: analgesics (paracetamol, NSAIDs, opioids), anti-emetics, 5-HT$_1$ agonists (e.g. sumatriptan), ergot alkaloids (e.g. ergotamine)

NEPHROLOGY

RENAL INVESTIGATIONS

- **Colour:** see Table 1.5

Table 1.5 Variations in urine colour

Colour	Cause
Clear light yellow	Normal
Lighter	Dilute
Darker	Concentrated
Red	Haematuria
White	Pyuria/phosphate crystals
Green	Amitriptyline/propofol
Black	Malignancy/haemolysis

- **Urine dipstick:** can detect albumin but not pathological proteins (i.e. Bence–Jones proteins or microalbuminuria)
- **Urine microscopy – casts:**
  - hyaline (not pathological, can be caused by diuretics)
  - red cell casts (glomerulonephritis, vasculitis)
  - white cell casts (tubulo-interstitial disease, acute pyelonephritis and some glomerulonephritis), epithelial cells (acute tubular necrosis [ATN], acute glomerulonephritis [AGN])
- **Urine microscopy – crystals:**
  - uric acid (+ ARF [acute renal failure] = tumour lysis syndrome)
  - calcium phosphate
  - oxalate
  - cystine (cystinuria)
- **Renal biopsy:**
  - *indication*: unexplained CRF (chronic renal failure) with normal/large kidneys, unexplained progressive renal impairment, nephrotic syndrome, renal impairment + proteinuria + haematuria ± systemic disorders, intrinsic ARF
  - *complications*: bleeding, localized bruising and pain, haematuria, sepsis, perforation of other organs
- **Glomerular filtration rate (GFR):** GFR is the volume of fluid filtered from the renal glomerular capillaries into Bowman's capsule per unit time. Clinically, this is often measured to determine renal function by the approximation:

$$\frac{\text{urine creatinine concentration} \times \text{urine volume (24 h)}}{\text{plasma creatinine concentration}}$$

  - normal GFR: male: 97–137 mL/min.; female: 88–128 mL/min
- **24-h protein:** normal <150 mg/day

GLOMERULONEPHRITIS (GN)

 Either primary or secondary (i.e. part of a systemic illness – Wegener's, SLE, diabetes, vasculitis)

P Inflammation of the glomeruli affecting both kidneys simultaneously
Histological classification:
- minimal change
- focal and segmental proliferative

- focal and segmental glomerulosclerosis
- mesangial proliferative GN (± IgA)
- crescentic GN
- membranous GN
- mesangiocapillary GN

S Features of either nephritic, nephrotic syndrome or non-specific i.e. weight loss, nausea and vomiting, anorexia, hiccups, pruritus, oliguria, nocturia (see Table 1.6)

Table 1.6 Presentations of renal disease

GN type	Renal failure	Nephrotic syndrome	Nephritic syndrome
Post-infection	++	–	+
Vasculitis	++	+	+
Crescentic mesangiocapillary	++	+	++
Membranous FSGS	+	++	++
Minimal change	+	++	+
Chronic infection	–	+	++

FSGS: focal segmental glomerulosclerosis

Ix *Bloods*: renal profile, blood film (haemolysis → haemolytic uraemic syndrome), arterial blood gases (ABG) (metabolic acidosis), C3 + C4 (low),
Auto-antibodies:
- ANA (SLE)
- cANCA (Wegener's granulomatosis)
- pANCA (polyarteritis nodosa)
- anti-GBM (Goodpasture's syndrome)
- antistreptolysin O (ASO) titres (post-streptococcal GN)
Urine: 24-h urine collection, protein and creatinine clearance, urine dipstick, urine MC&S
Radiology: USS renal tract
Histology: renal biopsy

Rx Treatment depends on underlying cause (i.e. steroids, immunosuppressants) Symptomatic; tight control of BP, diuretics; may need to consider dialysis/renal transplant

Cx CRF, end-stage renal failure

ACUTE NEPHRITIC SYNDROME

P Group of disorders that cause inflammation of the glomeruli

A Associated with post-group A β-haemolytic streptococcal sore throat (occurs about 2–3/52 later)
Other causes are haemolytic uraemic syndrome, IgA nephropathy, SLE

Sy Asymptomatic, occasionally oliguria, oedema, haematuria, arthralgia, myalgia, nausea, vomiting

Si Hypertension, oedema

Ix *Urine:* haematuria, mild proteinuria, urine microscopy for renal tubular cells, casts, red blood cells (RBCs), white blood cells (WBCs)
Bloods: FBC (↓ Hb, ↑ WBC), U&E, blood cultures

Immunology: ANA, ANCA, anti-GBM, C3, C4

Imaging: Renal USS, renal biopsy

Rx Bed rest, salt restriction, careful fluid monitoring, tight BP control, may need to consider steroids

Cx ARF, CRF, end-stage renal failure (ESRF)

Px Good: adults 60 per cent resolve, children 80–90 per cent

NEPHROTIC SYNDROME

P Classic triad of:
- proteinuria
- hypoalbuminaemia
- oedema (some add hyperlipidaemia)

A Long-standing diabetes mellitus (DM), GN (minimal change, membranous, focal segmental), amyloid (primary myeloma), autoimmune (SLE), drugs (gold, penicillamine)

Sy Weight gain, loss of appetite, nausea, vomiting, frothy urine, thrombosis

Si Mild hypertension, oedema (dependent sites plus face and hands)

Ix *Bloods:* renal profile, ↑ cholesterol, glucose, protein electrophoresis (myeloma), auto-antibodies (SLE, systemic vasculitis), albumin, clotting, hypogammaglobulinaemia

Urine: 24-h urine creatinine and protein, Bence–Jones protein

Imaging: renal USS/renal biopsy

Cx Hypercoagulability, hypercholesterolaemia, infection

Rx Diuretics, ACE inhibitors, anticoagulation, lipid-controlling agents

HAEMOLYTIC URAEMIC SYNDROME (HUS)

P Combination of haemolysis with red cell fragmentation, thrombocytopenia and acute renal failure

A Often post-infections, classically after pathogenic *E. coli O157*

Si As for acute renal failure

Ix Blood film, FBC, renal profile

Rx *Supportive:* fluids, blood / plasma transfusions

Dialysis

Cx Hypertension, chronic renal failure

ADULT POLYCYSTIC KIDNEY DISEASE (APKD)

P Numerous fluid-filled cysts in the kidneys

A Genetic disorder (autosomal dominant)

8–10 per cent of all ESRF

Presents in early adult life

Sy Dysuria, haematuria, loin pain (renal abscess), polyuria, nocturia, oliguria

Si ↑ BP, feature of renal disease, neurological signs secondary to subarachnoid haemorrhage (due to associated cerebral artery berry aneurysm)

Ix Anaemia, clotting, CT, USS

Rx *Patient education:* prognosis, genetic counselling

Medical: treat hypertension and infection

Surgery: transplantation

Cx Liver and pancreatic cysts, cerebral artery berry aneurysms, abnormal heart valves

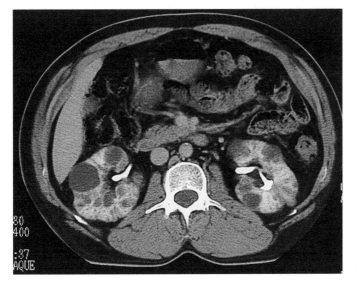

Figure 1.30 Adult polycystic kidney disease with well-defined low-density lesions in both kidneys

RENAL ARTERY STENOSIS

P Narrowing of the artery supplying the kidney
A Atherosclerosis, fibromuscular dysplasia, scar formation

Box 1.20 RISK FACTORS FOR RENAL ARTERY STENOSIS

- Carotid artery disease
- Coronary artery disease
- Smoking
- Peripheral vascular disease
- Diabetes
- Obesity

Sy Difficult to control BP, renal failure with ACE inhibitors
Si ↑ BP, renal bruit, flash pulmonary oedema
Ix *Imaging:* renal USS, MRA, renal Doppler USS, angiogram
Rx Control ↑ BP, renal balloon angioplasty and stenting
Cx Malignant hypertension, CRF, pulmonary oedema

GOODPASTURE'S SYNDROME

P Autoimmune: antibodies directed against Type IV collagen found in the glomerular and pulmonary alveolar basement membrane
A Commonly young males age 5–40 years (♂:♀ 6:1)
Rx Haematuria, proteinuria, renal failure, pulmonary haemorrhage, haemoptysis
Ix As for any cause of renal failure or pulmonary haemorrhage
Diagnostic markers are anti-GBM antibodies (present in >90 per cent)
Renal biopsy
Rx Plasmapheresis, steroids, immunosuppressants (cyclophosphamide/azathioprine), renal transplantation

URINARY TRACT INFECTION
See 'Urology' p. 202

RENAL FAILURE

ACUTE RENAL FAILURE (ARF)

P   Rapid potentially reversible decline in GFR over days to weeks

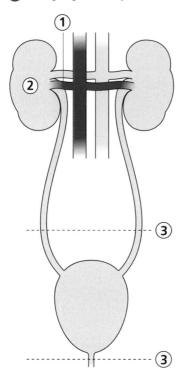

Figure 1.31 Causes of acute renal failure:

1 **Pre-renal:**
  hypovolaemia
  multiple organ failure
  rhabdomyolysis

2 **Renal:**
  acute GN
  acute allergic
     interstitial nephritis
  vasculitis
  acute tubular necrosis

3 **Post-renal:**
  prostatic hypertrophy
  blocked catheter
  extra-ureteric tumour
  retroperitoneal fibrosis

S   *General*: malaise, lethargy, myopathy
Genitourinary: oliguria, polyuria, nocturia
Dermatological: pruritus, rashes, purpura
Cardiovascular: ↑ BP, palpitations, pericarditis, oedema
GI: nausea, vomiting, hiccough
Respiratory: pulmonary oedema, Kussmaul's respiration
CNS: peripheral neuropathy, encephalopathy, fits

Ix   *Bloods:* FBC, U&E, blood film, blood cultures, ABG
Urine: MC&S
Imaging: CXR, renal USS

Rx   Treat underlying cause
Fluid monitoring (central venous pressure (CVP) line, accurate fluid input and output)
Indications for dialysis:
  – pulmonary oedema
  – $K^+ > 6.5$ mmol/L (refractory)

- pH < 7.2
- pericarditis
- encephalopathy

Box 1.21 TREATMENT OF HYPERKALAEMIA

- Calcium gluconate (decreases effect of potassium on heart)
- Dextrose and insulin infusion (transfers potassium intracellularly)
- Salbutamol nebulizer (transfers potassium intracellularly)
- Calcium resonium (removes potassium from body)

CHRONIC RENAL FAILURE (CRF)

 Abnormal GFR for >3/12

A GN, interstitial nephritis, reflux nephropathy, polycystic kidneys, DM, renovascular diseases, ↑ BP, obstructive uropathy

Sy Malaise, lethargy, nausea, vomiting, headache, hiccups, pruritus, SOB (shortness of breath, secondary to anaemia/pulmonary oedema)

Ix *Bloods*: chronic normochromic anaemia, hypocalcaemia + hyperphosphataemia (can develop hypercalcaemia due to tertiary hyperparathyroidism), metabolic acidosis, hyperkalaemia, low erythropoietin, low ferritin, ↓ activity of von Willebrand factor
Urine: MC&S, creatinine clearance (CrCl)
Imaging: renal USS

Rx Treat underlying cause, low-protein diet, BP control (reduces speed of deterioration), correct calcium, anaemia, acidosis, water retention.
Dialysis once CrCl < 20 mL/min

ENDOCRINOLOGY

DIABETES MELLITUS

P Chronic elevation of blood glucose

Ix Oral glucose tolerance test (OGTT): 75 g glucose to a fasting patient, measure baseline fasting glucose and then 2 h post glucose load (see Table 1.7)

Table 1.7 Diagnosis of diabetes and pre-diabetic conditions

	Normal	IFG	IGT	Diabetes
Fasting	≤6.0	6.1–6.9	< 7.0	≥7.0
2 h post-glucose load	< 7.8	< 7.8	7.8–11.0	≥11.1

IFG: impaired fasting glycaemia; IGT: impaired glucose tolerance

Cx *Macrovascular*: CVA, MI, peripheral vascular disease
Microvascular: retinopathy, nephropathy, neuropathy

TYPE 1 DIABETES

P Autoimmune destruction of the β cells in the islets of Langerhans in the pancreas leading to absolute insulin deficiency

A Twin studies: monozygotic concordance rate 45 per cent
Strong association with either HLA-DR3 or DR4 or both
Peak age of onset approximately 12 years

Sy Polyuria, polydipsia, weight loss ± ketoacidosis
Develops over days – months

Si Other features of autoimmune diseases

Ix *Blood*: U&E, FBC, glucose, antibodies
Immunology: anti-islet cell Ab (antibody), anti-GAD Ab
Urine: ketones, ABG

Rx *Supportive*: patient education
Glycaemic control: commence insulin, aim HbA_{1c} < 7 per cent, dietary advice
Complications surveillance: annual review (fundoscopy, feet examination →
neurological and vascular), check insulin sites, BP monitoring, monitor renal function, thyroid function

DIABETIC KETOACIDOSIS

A Precipitants include infections, MI, omitting insulin

Sy As above and nausea, vomiting, abdominal pain, tachypnoea (Kussmaul respiration secondary to metabolic acidosis)

Ix *Blood*: glucose, ABG (metabolic acidosis, large anion gap)
Urine: ketones ++++
Septic screen: CXR, urine, blood, stool cultures

Rx Insulin sliding scale, aggressive fluid replacement, monitor K^+ and replace, treat underlying cause

TYPE 2 DIABETES

P Combination of insulin resistance and inadequate production (β cell destruction) / impaired secretion of insulin (β cell dysfunction)

A Obesity, chronic pancreatitis, Cushing's syndrome
Twin studies: monozygotic concordance rate 90 per cent
Peak age of onset approx 50 years

Sy Often with complications of diabetes (e.g. peripheral vascular disease, CVA, MI), hyperosmolar non-ketotic coma (HONK), recurrent infection, pruritus

Si Increased BMI, retinopathy, peripheral neuropathy

Ix U&E, FBC, glucose, serum osmolality

Rx *Supportive*: patient education, dietary advice
Glycaemic control: initially treat with diet, if unsatisfactory glycaemic control consider oral hypoglycaemics, aim for HbA$_{1c}$ <7 per cent. Some patients may require insulin therapy
Complications surveillance: annual review (fundoscopy, feet examination $\rightarrow$ neurological and vascular), check insulin sites, BP monitoring, monitor renal function, thyroid function

Table 1.8 Oral agents used in Type 2 diabetes

Class	Example	Mechanism
Biguanides	Metformin	Improve sensitivity to insulin
Sulphonylureas	Gliclazide, glimepiride	Stimulate pancreatic insulin release
Thiazolidinediones	Rosiglitazone	Improve sensitivity to insulin
α-Glucosidase inhibitors	Acarbose	Prevent intestinal sugar absorption

HYPEROSMOLAR NON-KETOTIC COMA (HONK)

A Precipitant: infection, increased sugary intake, MI

Sy Polydipsia, polyuria, decreased consciousness, thrombosis

Ix $\uparrow$ Na$^+$, glucose (often >50 mmol/L), $\uparrow\uparrow$ osmolality

Rx CVP monitoring, fluid replacement, insulin, anticoagulation

Px Mortality 20–40 per cent

DIABETIC EYE DISEASE

See 'Ophthalmology' p. 206

HYPOGLYCAEMIA

A *SAIL*:
  – Sulphonylureas
  – Alcohol/Addison's
  – Insulinomas/Insulin/Infection (malaria, meningococcal),
  – Liver failure

Sy Cold sweat, tremor, irritability, loss of consciousness, collapse

Si Sweating, tachycardia, tremor, $\downarrow$ GCS (Glasgow Coma Score), fits

Ix Plasma glucose < 2.5 mmol/L
If non-diabetic: insulin + C-peptide + pro-insulin (during hypoglycaemic episode), LFT, ethanol levels, cortisol (short Synacthen test)

Rx Oral glucose (e.g. Lucozade), i.m. (intramuscular) glucagon (avoid in alcoholics), i.v. glucose

PITUITARY DISEASE

The pituitary consists of two main parts: anterior and posterior (see Table 1.9)

Table 1.9 Hormones of the pituitary gland

	Origin	Hormones
Anterior pituitary	Derived from Rathke's pouch	ACTH, TSH, LH, FSH, GH, prolactin
Posterior pituitary	Neural origin, nerve fibres originating in supraoptic and paraventricular nuclei in the hypothalamus	ADH, oxytocin

ACTH, adrenocorticotrophic hormone; TSH, thyroid-stimulating hormone; LH, luteinizing hormone; FSH, follicle-stimulating hormone; GH, growth hormone; ADH, antidiuretic hormone

HYPERPROLACTINAEMIA

P Elevated prolactin levels

A *Physiological*: pregnancy, breast feeding
Drugs: methyldopa, metoclopramide, haloperidol, oestrogen
Neoplasia: prolactinoma
Polycystic ovarian syndrome

Sy ♀: amenorrhoea, infertility, galactorrhoea (milk production)
♂: loss of libido, impotence, infertility, galactorrhoea
Pressure effects i.e. bitemporal hemianopia, hypopituitarism, cranial nerve palsies

Ix Full pituitary hormone profile, MRI pituitary, perimetry (visual field measurement)

Rx *Microprolactinoma* (<10 mm diameter): bromocriptine, cabergoline (dopamine agonists)
Macroprolactinoma (>10 mm diameter): trial of bromocriptine/cabergoline, if affecting visual fields then trans-sphenoidal surgery

Cx Untreated ↑ risk of osteoporosis

CUSHING'S SYNDROME

P Excess cortisol secretion

A See Box 1.22

Box 1.22 CAUSES OF CUSHING'S SYNDROME

- *Exogenous*: iatrogenic, steroids, pseudo Cushing's, excess alcohol, depression
- *ACTH dependent*: pituitary overproduction of ACTH stimulating adrenal gland to produce cortisol, Cushing's disease, ectopic ACTH secretion, small-cell lung cancer, carcinoid
- *ACTH independent*: autonomous cortisol secretion, adrenal adenoma/carcinoma/hyperplasia

---

Sy ↑ weight gain, poor wound healing, recurrent infections, depression, menstrual disturbances, low libido, hirsutism, headache, osteoporosis

(Si) Plethoric moon face, buffalo hump, angry purple abdominal striae, centripetal obesity, proximal myopathy, hirsutism, thin skin, easy bruising, hypertension, acne

(Ix) *24-h urinary collection*: free cortisol
Random blood cortisol: loss of circadian rhythm
Low-dose dexamethasone suppression test: confirm whether ACTH can be suppressed
High-dose dexamethasone suppression test: differentiate between pituitary and ectopic ACTH secretion
Once Cushing's syndrome is confirmed locate source

(Rx) Cushing's disease:
Surgery: trans-sphenoidal surgery
Cushing's syndrome:
Medical: metyrapone, ketoconazole
Surgery: adrenalectomy

(Cx) *Post-adrenalectomy*: Nelson's syndrome (↑ pigmentation, ↑ pituitary size), adrenal insufficiency
Post-transphenoidal surgery: hypopituitarism

(Px) If untreated poor

ACROMEGALY/GIGANTISM

(P) ↑ GH secretion

(Sy) Sweating, increase in size of hands and feet, headache, oligo/amenorrhoea, infertility

(Si) Macroglossia (enlarged tongue), prominent supra-orbital ridges, prognathism (prominent lower jaw), increased interdental spacing, doughy spade-like hands, carpal tunnel syndrome, bitemporal hemianopia, goitre, heart failure,

(Ix) Failure of suppression of GH in OGTT, insulin-like growth factor-1 (IGF-1), full pituitary hormone profile, MRI pituitary, visual fields, fasting glucose

(Rx) *Medical*: cabergoline, octreotide (somatostatin analogue)
Surgery: transphenoidal surgery ± radiotherapy

(Cx) Diabetes mellitus, heart failure, osteoporosis, obstructive sleep apnoea, ↑ risk of colonic polyps and colonic carcinoma (hence patients require colonoscopy every 3 years), hypopituitarism

(Px) If untreated mortality is high

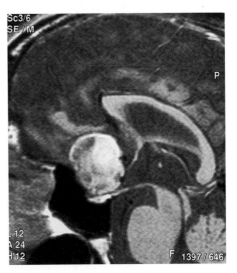

Figure 1.32 Sagittal MRI section shows a large pituitary tumour of mixed signal

THYROID DISEASE

THYROTOXICOSIS

(P) Excess thyroxine production

(A) Viral thyroiditis, hyperthyroidism (toxic adenoma, toxic nodule in a MNG, Graves' disease), drugs (amiodarone, lithium), struma ovarii (rare ovarian cancer)
Most commonly affects young females

(Sy) Weight loss, increased appetite, diarrhoea, palpitations, tremor, agitation, psychosis, heat intolerance, increased sweating, SOB, oligomenorrhoea

(Si) Tachycardia, warm, sweaty, fine tremor, lid lag, lid retraction, palmar erythema, hair loss, myopathy, goitre
Specific for Graves': thyroid acropachy (like clubbing), pre-tibial myxoedema
Eye signs: peri-orbital oedema, exophthalmos, proptosis, ophthalmoplegia

(Ix) $\uparrow$ thyroxine (T_4), $\uparrow$ tri-iodothyronine (T_3), $\downarrow$ thyroid-stimulating hormone (TSH), TSH receptor antibody (specific for Graves'), ^{99m}Tc uptake scan, ESR

(Rx) *Medical*: antithyroid drugs e.g. carbimazole often first-line treatment, β-blockers (e.g. propranolol) for symptom relief
Radiation ablation: radio-iodine only for patients over 45 years
Surgery: partial thyroidectomy (see p. 150 for details)
Viral thyroiditis: analgesia, steroids

(Cx) Heart failure, osteoporosis. Small incidence of agranulocytosis with carbimazole (measure FBC regularly)

HYPOTHYROIDISM

(P) Deficiency of T_4

(A) See Box 1.23

Box 1.23 CAUSES OF HYPOTHYROIDISM

- *Autoimmune*: Hashimoto's thyroiditis
- *Dietary*: iodine deficiency
- *Congenital*
- *Panhypopituitarism*
- *Iatrogenic*: post-surgery/radio-iodine
- *Drugs*: amiodarone, lithium

(Sy) Fatigue, lethargy, cold intolerance, constipation, weight gain, carpal tunnel syndrome, menorrhagia, oligo/amenorrhoea, low mood, dry skin, hair loss

(Si) Peri-orbital puffiness, loss of lateral third of eyebrows, cerebellar signs, slow reflexes

(Ix) TFTs ($\uparrow$ TSH, $\downarrow$ T_4)

(Rx) Replacement with levothyroxine

(Cx) If untreated can result in myxoedema coma

PARATHYROID GLAND DISORDERS

Classically the parathyroids are four glands lying behind the thyroid (number and position vary). They secrete parathyroid hormone (PTH) which $\uparrow Ca^{2+}$ and $\downarrow PO_4^{3-}$

HYPERCALCAEMIA

 Most commonly bone metastasis (lung, breast) and hyperparathyroidism
Myeloma, sarcoidosis, thyrotoxicosis, FHH (familial hypocalciuric hypercalcaemia)

 Bones, stones, moans and groans (see Box 1.24); polydipsia, polyuria

 Bloods: Ca^{2+}, albumin, ALP, PTH, PTH-related peptide (PTHrP), vitamin D, ACE, TFTs, tumour markers, urinary Ca^{2+}
ECG: shortened QT interval
Imaging: bone scan, sestamibi scan, CXR, mammogram (if suspicious of breast cancer)

 Aggressive fluid rehydration, then loop diuretics
Treat underlying cause:
- *hyperparathyroidism*: surgery (if Ca^{2+} >3 mmol/L + symptomatic or renal stones), bisphosphonates (e.g. alendronate)
- *bone metastases*: bisphosphonates
- *sarcoidosis*: steroids

PRIMARY HYPERPARATHYROIDISM

 85 per cent due to solitary parathyroid adenoma, 15 per cent due to hyperplasia, <1 per cent carcinoma

Associated with multiple endocrine neoplasia (MEN) syndromes I and II

50 per cent asymptomatic. For the other 50 per cent remember the aide mémoire in Box 1.24

Box 1.24 FEATURES OF HYPERCALCAEMIA

- Painful bones (± fractures)
- Renal stones
- Abdominal groans (abdominal pain)
- Psychic moans (depression)

 Bloods $\uparrow$ PTH in the setting of $\uparrow Ca^{2+}$
Raised 24-h urinary calcium
Sestamibi nuclear medicine scan used to identify position of adenomas

 High fluid intake (prevent renal stone formation)
Surgical resection indicated if symptoms are significant

Risk of transient hypocalcaemia post-operatively

SECONDARY HYPERPARATHYROIDISM

Raised PTH in response to low calcium (e.g. renal failure, vitamin D deficiency)

TERTIARY HYPERPARATHYROIDISM

P   Prolonged secondary hyperparathyroidism results in autonomous excessive production of PTH and resultant hypercalcaemia

HYPOCALCAEMIA

A   Hypoalbuminaemia, hypomagnesaemia, hyperphosphataemia, medication effects, surgical effects, PTH deficiency or resistance, and vitamin D deficiency or resistance, acute pancreatitis

Sy   Muscle ache, pins and needles, tetany, bony pain

Si   Chvostek's sign, Trousseau's sign, arrhythmias

Ix Ca^{2+}, PO_4, ALP, vitamin D, PTH, Mg^{2+}, U&E

Rx   Calcium replacement

INFORMATION BOX: SIGNS OF HYPOCALCAEMIA

- *Chvostek's sign*: tap over the facial nerve about 2 cm anterior to the tragus of the ear (twitching first at the angle of the mouth, then by the nose, the eye, and the facial muscles)
- *Trousseau's sign*: inflation of a blood pressure cuff above the systolic pressure causes local ulnar and median nerve ischaemia, resulting in carpal spasm

---

PRIMARY HYPOPARATHYROIDISM

A   Most commonly iatrogenic: inadvertent removal during thyroidectomy or post-radiation

Sy   Tetany, depression, paraesthesiae

Si   Chvostek's sign, Trousseau's sign

Ix   *Bloods:* $\downarrow Ca^{2+}$ and $\uparrow PO_4^{3-}$

Rx   Calcium and vitamin D supplementation

PSEUDOHYPOPARATHYROIDISM

P   Cells resistant to PTH

Si   Pixie face, short metacarpals and metatarsals

PSEUDOPSEUDOHYPOPARATHYROIDISM

P   Same morphological features as pseudohypoparathyroidism but normal biochemical profile

ADRENAL GLAND DISORDERS

PHAEOCHROMOCYTOMA

P   Tumour of the adrenal medulla secreting noradrenaline and adrenaline
90 per cent benign, unilateral
10 per cent malignant, multiple

A   Can be part of MEN IIA/B

Sy   Episodic flushing, palpitations, sweating, headache

Si   Hypertension, pallor

Ix 24-h urinary catecholamines ×3
   If positive: MRI adrenal, ^{131}I-MIBG nuclear medicine scan, exclude MEN II
Rx *Medical*: phenoxybenzamine, needs adequate α blockade prior to β blockade
   Surgery: laparoscopic adrenalectomy

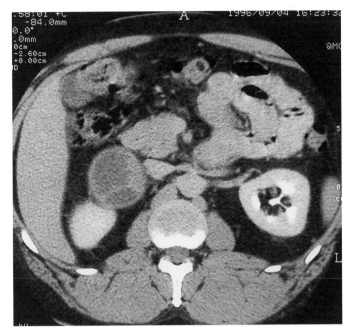

Figure 1.33
Phaeochromocytoma: a well-circumscribed mass in the right adrenal gland

CONN'S SYNDROME

P 60 per cent unilateral adrenocortical adenoma producing excess aldosterone
   40 per cent bilateral adrenal hyperplasia
Si ↑BP
Ix *Blood*: hypokalaemia, hypernatraemia, metabolic alkalosis, aldosterone/renin ratio
   Radiology: iodine ^{131}I iodocholesterol scanning, CT/MRI
Rx *Medical*: spironolactone (aldosterone antagonist)
   Surgery: resection

ADDISON'S DISEASE

P Destruction of the adrenal cortices, resulting in steroid and mineralocorticoid deficiency
A Autoimmune (90 per cent), TB, metastasis
Sy Weight loss, abdominal pain, lethargy, malaise, nausea, vomiting, diarrhoea
Si Hyperpigmentation, postural hypotension, vitiligo
Ix Hyponatraemia, short Synacthen, exclude other autoimmune conditions
Rx Hydrocortisone (to replace steroid), fludrocortisone (to replace mineralocorticoid)

CONGENITAL ADRENAL HYPERPLASIA

 Autosomal recessive condition resulting in partial to complete deficiency of an enzyme necessary for the synthesis of aldosterone or cortisol production in the adrenal gland

Si *21-hydroxylase deficiency*: most common, can present with either salt-losing crisis or female virilization
11β-hydroxylase deficiency: presents with female virilization, hypertension
17α-hydroxylase deficiency: presents with male undervirilization, hypokalaemia, hypertension

Rx Long-term replacement with glucocorticoid or aldosterone or both

DISORDERS OF WATER REGULATION

DIABETES INSIPIDUS (DI)

P Inability of the kidneys to conserve water, which leads to frequent urination and pronounced thirst

Table 1.10 The causes of diabetes insipidus

	Pathology	Causes
Cranial	Failure of posterior pituitary to produce vasopressin	Idiopathic Brain tumours Surgery Head trauma Meningitis
Nephrogenic	Failure of kidneys to respond to vasopressin	Hypercalcaemia Hypokalaemia Demeclocycline, lithium Chronic renal disease

Sy Polyuria, polydipsia
Ix Urine/plasma osmolality
Water deprivation test (in cranial DI urine osmolality will ↑ when given desmopressin, no response in nephrogenic DI)
 Cranial: desmopressin (ADH analogue)
Nephrogenic: treat underlying cause, thiazide diuretics (paradoxical effect)

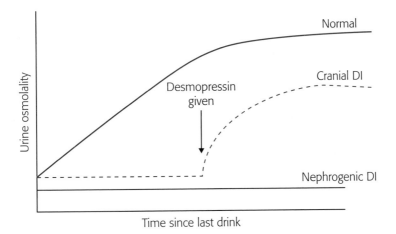

Figure 1.34 Water deprivation test

SYNDROME OF INAPPROPRIATE ANTIDIURETIC HORMONE (SIADH)

Ⓟ   ADH (vasopressin) causes water retention by increasing the permeability of the nephrons
ADH is produced by the hypothalamus and released from the posterior pituitary gland

---

Box 1.25 CAUSES OF THE SYNDROME OF INAPPROPRIATE ADH

- *CNS disorders*: meningitis, encephalitis, tumour, CVA, subarachnoid haemorrhage (SAH)
- *Pulmonary*: TB, empyema, asthma, COPD
- *Malignancy*: lung, pancreas, lymphoma
- *Drugs*: antidepressants, carbamazepine, cyclophosphamide, diuretics, neuroleptics, barbiturates

---

ⓈⓎ   Acute anorexia, nausea and vomiting
Na^+ *110–115 mmol/L*: headache, irritability, disorientation and weakness
Na^+ *<110 mmol/L*: delirium, psychosis, ataxia, tremor
Ⓢⓘ   Euvolaemic, papilloedema, severe myoclonus
Ⓘⓧ   ↓ Na^+, ↓ serum osmolality, inappropriately dilute urine (250–1400 mosmol/kg), TFTs, 09:00 cortisol/short Synacthen, CT head
Ⓡⓧ   Fluid restriction, correct Na^+ at a rate < 12 mEq/L/day
Ⓒⓧ   If Na^+ increased too rapidly: central pontine myelinolysis (usually fatal)

RHEUMATOLOGY

RHEUMATOID ARTHRITIS (RA)

(P) Systemic autoimmune disorder affecting the synovial joints with extra-articular manifestations

(A) Prevalence is 1–3 per cent, ♀ > ♂, peak age of onset 40 years

(Sy) Joint pain exacerbated by movement, morning stiffness, joint swelling
Extra-articular manifestations (see below)
Systemic: fever (mild), anorexia, malaise, weight loss, lethargy

(Si) Joints: swollen, warm, tender joints,
Joint deformities (swan neck, boutonnière), subluxation
Lymphadenopathy, splenomegaly
Rheumatoid nodules
Muscle weakness, evidence of amyloidosis and vasculitis

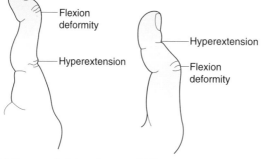

(a) **Swan neck deformity**   (b) **Boutonnière**

Figure 1.35 Joint deformities in rheumatoid arthritis (figure 1.35(a) adapted with kind permission from Model D, *Making Sense of Clinical Examination of the Adult Patient*, Great Britain: Hodder Arnold, 2006)

Box 1.26 DIAGNOSTIC CRITERIA FOR RHEUMATOID ARTHRITIS

(need 4 out of 7 – 'RF RISES')
- **R**heumatoid factor
- **F**inger/hand joint involvement
- **R**heumatoid nodules
- **I**nvolvement of 3 or more joints
- **S**tiffness – early morning
- **E**rosions/decalcification on x-rays
- **S**ymmetrical arthritis

(Ix) *Bloods*: ESR + CRP (degree of synovial inflammation), anaemia of chronic disease, low albumin (correlates directly with disease severity)
Immunology: rheumatoid factor (RhF), anti-CCP (cyclic citrullinated peptide) Ab (may be a better predictor of progression to erosive joint disease than titres of RhF),
X-rays: soft tissue swelling, joint space narrowing, peri-articular osteoporosis, bony erosions, deformities, atlanto-axial subluxation
Synovial fluid: ↑WBC, ↑protein

(Rx) *Goals*: pain relief, protection of remaining articular structure, maintenance of function

Patient education: encourage rest alternating with exercise
Physiotherapy and occupational therapy
Medical: analgesics, NSAIDs, glucocorticoids, DMARDs (disease-modifying antirheumatic drugs)

Table 1.11 Disease-modifying antirheumatic drugs

Non-biological	Biological
Methotrexate	Soluble interleukin-1 (IL-1) receptor therapy (anakinra)
Hydroxychloroquine	Tumour necrosis factor inhibitors (e.g. etanercept, infliximab)
Sulfasalazine	Cytotoxic agents (azathioprine, cyclophosphamide, and ciclosporin A)
Leflunomide	
Penicillamine	
Gold	

Cx *Respiratory*: pulmonary nodules, fibrosing alveolitis, pleural effusion, Caplan's syndrome (rheumatoid arthritis in coal miners with pneumoconiosis) and bronchiolitis obliterans
CVS (cardiovascular system): endocarditis, pericarditis, myocarditis, nodules
CNS: entrapment neuropathies, peripheral neuropathy
Eyes: episcleritis, scleritis, kerato-conjunctivitis, scleromalacia
Others: Felty's syndrome (RhF +ve, splenomegaly and neutropenia)

Px Variable. Poor prognostic factors include systemic involvement, insidious onset, rheumatoid nodules, RhF > 1:512, persistent activity for >12 months and early bone erosions

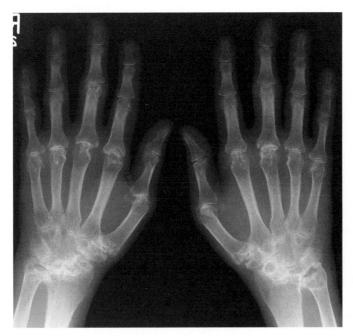

Figure 1.36 Rheumatoid arthritis: erosions at the metacarpophalangeal joints; note peri-articular soft tissue swelling and the severe changes at both wrists

REITER'S SYNDROME

(P) Triad of:
  – seronegative oligoarticular asymmetrical arthritis
  – urethritis and/or cervicitis
  – conjunctivitis

(A) Male predisposition, age 16–25 years, associated with human leucocyte antigen (HLA) B27
Triggered by *Chlamydia, Salmonella, Shigella, Yersinia* and *Campylobacter*

(Sy) Malaise, fever, arthritis, urethritis, conjunctivitis

(Si) Joint swelling and pain, dactylitis (sausage finger/toe), circinate balanitis, keratoderma blennorrhagica (papules on palms, soles and glans penis)

(Ix) No specific tests. ↑CRP and ESR, –ve RhF and synovial fluid, urinalysis, culture – urine, stool, synovial fluid, high urethral/vaginal swab and serology for *Chlamydia*

(Rx) Bed rest, intra-articular steroids, NSAIDs, for recurrent or chronic symptoms consider DMARDs

(Px) 33 per cent have recurrent/sustained disease
15–22 per cent permanent disability

SEPTIC ARTHRITIS

(P) Can occur due to either haematological spread, direct spread from an adjacent source, or through direct introduction of the organism via trauma/instrumentation

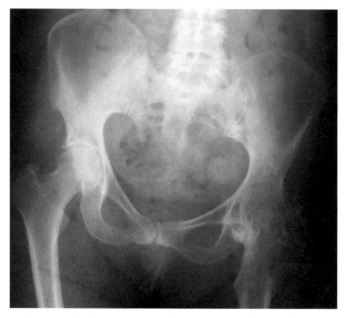

Figure 1.37 Complete ankylosis of the hip joint following a septic arthritis

(A) Bacterial causes include *S. aureus, S. pyogenes, N. gonorrhoea* (young adults), *Salmonella* (sickle cell)

(S) Fever, warm, red, swollen, painful joint, may also be an erythematous rash

(Ix) *Bloods*: ↑WBC, uric acid (exclude gout), antibodies (exclude RA), cultures
Synovial fluid: cloudy, ↑leucocytes, culture
Urine: MC&S
Microbiology: urethral, cervical and anorectal swabs

X-rays: soft tissue swelling, joint distension, later juxta-articular osteoporosis, periosteal elevation, joint space narrowing, bony erosions and possible osteomyelitis

Rx Physiotherapy, analgesia, antibiotics, aspiration and drainage

Cx Joint destruction

SYSTEMIC LUPUS ERYTHEMATOSUS (SLE)

P Multisystemic disease in which antibodies and immune complexes may cause cellular and tissue damage

A Most common in African–Caribbean women aged 25–35 years
Concordance in twins, plus familial tendency

Box 1.27 DIAGNOSTIC CRITERIA FOR SLE

(need 4 out of 11 – 'ORDER HIS ANA')
- **O**ral ulcers
- **R**ash (malar)
- **D**iscoid rash
- **E**xaggerated photosensitivity
- **R**enal disease
- **H**aematological abnormality
- **I**mmunological abnormality
- **S**erositis
- **A**rthralgia
- **N**eurological disease
- **A**NA

Sy Malaise, fever, arthralgia

Si Malar 'butterfly' rash, discoid lupus, mucosal ulcers, vasculitic rash, symmetrical arthritis, Raynaud's, Sjögren's, episcleritis, retinal infarcts, optic neuritis

Ix *Bloods*: Coombs' +ve haemolytic anaemia, neutropenia, lymphocytopenia, thrombocytopenia, ↑ESR, → CRP, renal profile,
Antibodies: ANA, anti-dsDNA, anti-smRNA, antiphospholipid Ab, anti-Ro/La, ↓C3 + C4

Rx *Minor symptoms*: NSAIDs, anti-malarials, low-dose steroids
Major symptoms: Steroids and immunosuppressants

Cx *Renal*: 50 per cent can develop lupus nephritis
CNS: psychosis, stroke, fits
CVS: pericarditis, myocarditis, Libman–Sacks endocarditis (autoimmune)
Respiratory system: pleural effusion, pneumonitis, ARDS

ANTIPHOSPHOLIPID SYNDROME

A Can be primary or associated with other autoimmune conditions e.g. SLE

Sy Recurrent venous/arterial thrombosis (i.e. CVA, Budd–Chiari syndrome, DVT)
Recurrent spontaneous miscarriages

Si Livedo reticularis, purpura, splinter haemorrhages, valvular heart disease

Ix ↑activated partial thromboplastin time (APTT), thrombocytopenia, haemolytic anaemia, anticardiolipin Ab, lupus anticoagulant

Rx Aspirin 75 mg daily; if the patient develops a thromboembolic event, warfarin anticoagulation

SYSTEMIC SCLEROSIS

(A) Associated with malignancy

(P) Multisystemic connective tissue disease causing inflammation, fibrosis and vascular damage to the skin and internal organs
Syndromes:
- limited cutaneous systemic sclerosis (skin involvement distally, systemic involvement occurs late and is rare, anticentromere antibody (ACA) +ve 70 per cent)
- diffuse cutaneous systemic sclerosis (early systemic involvement, Scl-70 (topoisomerase) antibody +ve 30 per cent)

(Sy) Pruritus, Raynaud's, dysphagia, nausea, vomiting, abdominal pain, diarrhoea, faecal incontinence, SOB, non-productive cough, palpitations, weakness, arthralgia, dry eyes

(Si) *Major features*: centrally located skin sclerosis – arms, face ± neck.
Minor features: sclerodactyly (tight skin over fingers), erosions, atrophy of the fingertips, and bilateral lung fibrosis

(Ix) *Bloods*: $\uparrow$ MCV, $\rightarrow$ ESR, $\uparrow$ urea + creatinine (if there is renal involvement), $\uparrow$ CK (mild), $\uparrow$ Ig, ANA (90 per cent),
Imaging: CXR/CT of the chest (linear/nodular interstitial fibrosis)

(Rx) Patient education + counselling
Physiotherapy + occupational therapy (OT)
Drugs:
- *Raynaud's*: Ca^{2+} channel antagonists (nifedipine), prostaglandin infusions
- *GI symptoms*: antacids, H_2 blockers, laxatives
- *myositis*: corticosteroids
- *renal crisis*: ACE inhibitors
- *cardiac*: anti-arrhythmics
- *early stage diffuse form*: immunosuppressants
- *late stage*: antifibrotics e.g. penicillamine

PSORIATIC ARTHRITIS

(P) Chronic seronegative inflammatory arthritis associated with psoriasis

(A) 10 per cent of patients with psoriasis develop arthritis, mean age of onset 40–50 years
Associated with HLA-B27

(Sy) Asymmetric large joint oligoarthritis, axial arthritis, asymmetrical sacroiliitis, peripheral small joint arthritis, distal interphalangeal joint (DIP) arthritis and arthritis mutilans; stiffness

(Si) Enthesitis, dactylitis, psoriasis,
Nail changes: onycholysis, transverse ridging, nail pitting

(Ix) *Bloods*: $\uparrow$ ESR, RhF –ve, ANA –ve
Synovial fluid: –ve
Imaging: X-rays: para-marginal erosions, fluffy periosteal bone formation, bony ankylosis, asymmetric sacroiliitis

(Rx) Physiotherapy, occupational therapy, NSAIDs, DMARDs

ANKYLOSING SPONDYLITIS

(P) Chronic seronegative disease of unknown aetiology, resulting in inflammation of multiple articular and para-articular structures – bony ankylosis

(A) Associated with HLA-B27 (up to 95 per cent of patients)
Onset occurs in late teens/ early adulthood, ♂ > ♀

(Sy) Lower back pain and early morning stiffness, enthesitis, anterior uveitis, pain in hips, buttocks and shoulders

(Si) Tenderness over the sacroiliac joint, ↓ anterior flexion of the lumbar spine, thoracic spinal fusion, ↓ lateral spine flexion, ↓ chest expansion, aortic regurgitation, apical lung fibrosis

(Ix) *Bloods*: chronic anaemia, RhF –ve, ↑ ESR
Imaging: X-ray – sacroiliitis, juxta-articular sclerosis, syndesmophyte formation, marginal erosion, fusion of adjacent vertebrae *(bamboo spine)*, disk calcification, pseudarthrosis; MRI

(Rx) Physiotherapy, occupational therapy, NSAIDs, DMARDs

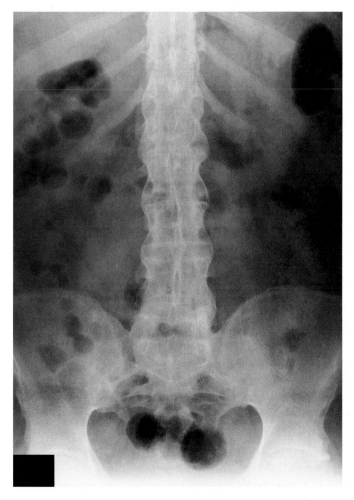

Figure 1.38 Ankylosing spondylitis: 'bamboo spine' with fusion of the sacroiliac joints

MYOSITIS: POLYMYOSITIS/DERMATOMYOSITIS

(P) Inflammatory disease of skeletal muscle of unknown aetiology
Dermatomyositis = polymyositis (muscle involvement only) + skin involvement

(A) Primary or secondary associated with autoimmune rheumatic disease or malignancy

(Sy) Progressive proximal muscle weakness, myalgia, dysphagia, SOB

(Si) Dermatomyositis: periorbital oedema, heliotrope rash, Gottron's papules (erythematous scaly lesions affecting the dorsum of the hands)

(Ix) ↑CK, ANA, Anti-Jo1 Ab, exclude malignancy, EMG, muscle biopsy

(Rx) *Medical*: high-dose glucocorticoids, azathioprine/methotrexate, immunoglobulin
Physiotherapy

SJÖGREN'S SYNDROME

(P) Autoimmune disease that causes progressive destruction of exocrine glands and polyarthritis

(A) Primary or associated with other autoimmune rheumatic diseases
♀ > ♂

(Sy) Oral soreness, eye dryness, mild relapsing non-erosive polyarthritis

(Si) Angular stomatitis, eye redness, xeroderma

(Ix) ESR, RhF, ANA, anti-Ro, anti-La, lip biopsy

(Rx) *Supportive*: artificial tears, mouthwash

(Cx) Acute/chronic pancreatitis, nephrogenic DI, renal tubular acidosis, interstitial nephritis, glomerulonephritis, neuropathy (peripheral sensory, sensorimotor, cranial)

POLYARTERITIS NODOSA

(P) Necrotizing vasculitis of small and medium-sized vessels

(A) Associated with HBV, hepatitis C, CMV, HIV

(Sy) Weight loss, fever, malaise, myalgia, polyarthritis, rapid renal failure

(Si) ↑BP, acute abdomen, mononeuritis multiplex, fever, livedo reticularis,

(Ix) *Bloods*: FBC (neutrophilia), U&E ↑ESR, ↑ALP, ANCA, viral serology, blood cultures
Urine: microscopy, creatinine clearance
Imaging: CXR, arteriography (multiple small aneurysms)

(Rx) Corticosteroids, cytotoxic drugs

(Px) Worse prognosis with heavy proteinuria, renal insufficiency (creatinine >140 mmol/L), cardiomyopathy, GI manifestations, CNS involvement

POLYMYALGIA RHEUMATICA

(A) Older patients, ♀:♂ 2:1

(Sy) Bilateral proximal muscle stiffness and ache, systemic features (weight loss, fever, malaise)

(Si) Normal muscle power

(Ix) FBC (normocytic normochromic anaemia), ↑ESR

(Rx) Low-dose corticosteroids, often for months/years

WEGENER'S GRANULOMATOSIS

(P) Systemic vascular disease characterized by necrotizing granulomas in the respiratory tract and focal necrotizing glomerulonephritis

(Sy) Cough, pleurisy, SOB, haemoptysis, general malaise, haematuria, arthralgia, purulent/bloody nasal discharge

(Si) Purpura, oral ulceration, pleural effusion, conjunctivitis

(Ix) *Bloods:* FBC (leucocytosis, thrombocytosis), cANCA
Blood film: schistocytes, Burr cells
Urine: proteinuria, haematuria, red cell casts
Imaging: CXR – migrating rounded opacities ± cavitation, pleural effusions, infiltrates; CT scan
Biopsy: affected organs show granulomatous changes

(Rx) Immunosuppressants, corticosteroids

TEMPORAL ARTERITIS

(P) Systemic inflammatory vasculitis of unknown aetiology that affects medium- and large-sized arteries

(A) Mostly in those aged over 50 years; ♀ > ♂

(Sy) Headache, malaise, transient visual disturbance, blindness, fever, lethargy, jaw claudication

(Si) Tender, non-pulsatile temporal arteries, proximal muscle tenderness

(Ix) ↑ESR, temporal artery biopsy

(Rx) High-dose glucocorticoids – do not wait for biopsy

(Cx) Blindness, aortitis, aortic dissection/aneurysm

TAKAYASU'S ARTERITIS

(P) Chronic, progressive, inflammatory, occlusive disease of the aorta and its branches (i.e. large blood vessels)

(A) Young females, 15–35 years

(Sy) Systemic illness + tenderness over palpable arteries, bruits, loss of pulses, claudication pain

(Rx) Steroids ± immunosuppressants; angioplasty/surgical repair for stenosed vessels

(Cx) Renovascular hypertension

BEHÇET'S DISEASE

(P) Chronic autoimmune vasculitis causing characteristic skin, eye and mucosal lesions

(A) ♂ > ♀, common in Turkey, Iran

(S) *Major criteria*: recurrent aphthous stomatitis, sterile pustules at site of skin trauma (pathergy test), uveitis, genital ulceration
Minor criteria: inflammatory large joint arthritis, intestinal ulceration, meningoencephalitis, epididymitis, thrombophlebitis

(Rx) Steroids/ciclosporin A

GOUT

(P) Uric acid arthropathy

(A) ♂ > ♀

↑dietary purine intake, alcohol, ↑cell turnover (i.e. malignancy), low-dose aspirin, diuretics, inherited enzyme deficiencies

(Sy) *Acute*: monoarthritis, severe pain lasting 7–10 days, most commonly first metatarsophalangeal joint (podagra)

Chronic: gouty tophi on pinnae, hands ± polyarthritis

(Ix) Uric acid levels, synovial fluid microscopy for crystals (negatively birefringent), *Imaging*: X-ray: cortical erosions, sclerotic margins

(Rx) Dietary changes, decrease alcohol intake, NSAIDs, colchicine, allopurinol (to prevent recurrence, but avoid in acute attack)

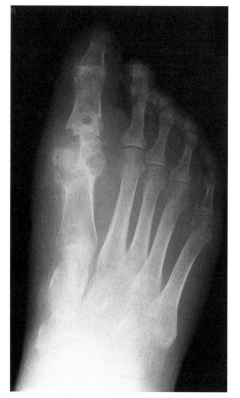

Figure 1.39 Gout of the big toe with soft tissue swelling and sharp well-defined erosions

PSEUDOGOUT

(P) Calcium pyrophosphate arthropathy

(A) Primary or secondary to hyperparathyroidism, haemochromatosis, diabetes, Wilson's disease, hypothyroidism

(Ix) *Imaging*: X-ray shows chondrocalcinosis

Joint aspiration: positively birefringent crystals

(Rx) NSAIDs, colchicine

PAGET'S DISEASE

 P Chronic disorder of bone remodelling leading to disorganized structure of woven and lamellar bone

A ♂ > ♀, >70 years

Sy Pain at affected site, most commonly pelvis, lumbar spine, femur; hearing loss due to VIIIth nerve compression

Si Sabre tibia, ↑ warmth over affected area, ↑ head size ± frontal bossing, conductive/sensory hearing loss, basilar invagination

Ix *Bloods*: ↑ ALP, → Ca^{2+},
Imaging: X-ray: expansion + deformity of affected long bones with mixed osteolytic + sclerotic areas

Rx Bisphosphonates (e.g. alendronate) for active disease, calcitonin for severe pain/extensive lytic disease

Cx Osteosarcoma, fractures, high-output cardiac failure, hypercalcaemia, secondary immobility

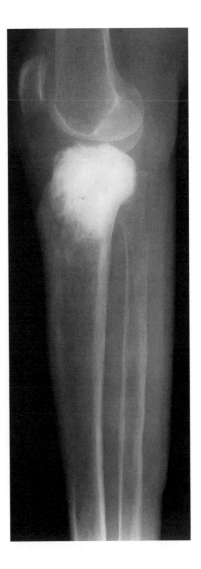

Figure 1.40 Paget's disease: tibial bowing, cortical thickening and abnormal modelling

OSTEOPOROSIS

P   ↓ quantity of bone/unit volume, resulting in decreased skeletal strength

A   ♀ > ♂, occurs in up to 30 per cent of post-menopausal women

Idiopathic or secondary to endocrine disorders (e.g. Cushing's syndrome, thyrotoxicosis, osteomalacia), corticosteroids, chronic renal failure, multiple myeloma, alcoholism, hereditary

Sy   Fractures

Ix   DEXA (dual-energy X-ray absorptiometry), bone density scan

Rx   Exclude secondary causes, prevention with exercise, ↑ dietary intake, stop smoking, Ca^{2+} supplements (e.g. Calcichew), bisphosphonates

OSTEOMALACIA

P   Heterogeneous disorders characterized by defective bone mineralization of newly synthesized bone

A   Most common in children/elderly

Causes: dietary, malabsorption, chronic pancreatitis, CRF (unable to hydroxylate vitamin D), Fanconi syndrome, phenytoin

Si   Bony deformities, bone pain + tenderness, proximal myopathy

Ix   *Bloods*: ↓ Ca^{2+}, ↓ PO_4, ↑ ALP, ↑ PTH, ↓ 25-OH vitamin D

Imaging: X-ray: Looser's zones (radiolucent areas occurring at right angles to the cortex)

Rx   Vitamin D replacement

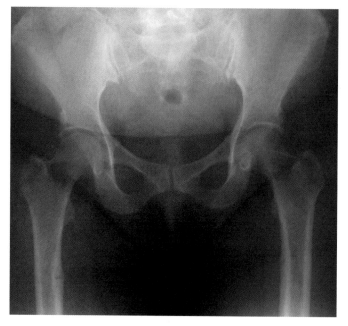

Figure 1.41

Osteomalacia: Looser's zones in the medial aspects of both femora

HAEMATOLOGY

ANAEMIA

P ↓ Hb, classified according to either aetiology or red cell morphology
Sy Lethargy, SOB, palpitations, chest pains, headaches
Si Pallor, systolic flow murmur, specific signs to the underlying condition

MICROCYTIC ANAEMIA (↓ MEAN CORPUSCULAR VOLUME [MCV])

IRON DEFICIENCY ANAEMIA

P Daily requirements, females 1.5 mg/day, pregnancy 7.5 mg/day, men 1 mg/day
Iron is absorbed from the small intestine, transported in the blood via transferrin and stored attached to ferritin
A Chronic blood loss (GI, menstruation), malabsorption, GI malignancy (in the elderly, assume iron deficiency anaemia is due to colon cancer until proven otherwise)
Si Koilonychia, sore tongue, angular stomatitis, Plummer–Vinson syndrome (dysphagia secondary to oesophageal web), painless gastritis
Ix FBC, ↓ ferritin, ↓ serum iron, ↑ TIBC, ↓ transferrin saturation, OGD, colonoscopy/barium enema
Rx Diagnose and treat underlying cause
Ferrous sulphate until Hb and MCV normal
Blood transfusion only if patient is symptomatic or a cardiac patient (keep Hb >10 g/dL)

β THALASSAEMIA

A Most common autosomal recessive inherited haematological disorder
Commonest in Mediterranean, Middle East, Asia
P ↓ β-globin production, leading to chronic anaemia
Si *Homozygotes*: failure to thrive, severe anaemia, splenomegaly, bone hypertrophy (secondary to extramedullary haemopoiesis)
Heterozygotes: usually asymptomatic, mildly anaemic, ↓↓ MCV
Ix Hb electrophoresis, blood film
Rx Repeated blood transfusions
Cx Secondary haemosiderosis, from repeated blood transfusions, endocrine disease

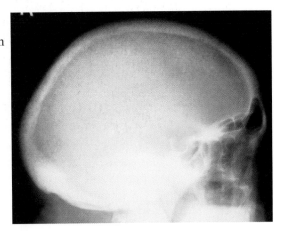

Figure 1.42 Expansion of the diploic space in thalassaemia due to extramedullary haemopoiesis

SICKLE CELL DISEASE

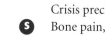

- **A** Autosomal recessive genetic disease due to haemoglobin chain mutation
- **P** Abnormal haemoglobin (HbS) has tendency to become rigid and sickle, causing occlusion of small vessels ('sickle cell crisis')
  Crisis precipitated by infection, dehydration, hypoxia, cold
- **S** Bone pain, pleuritic pain, priapism, jaundice and pigment gallstones secondary to chronic haemolysis, failure to thrive

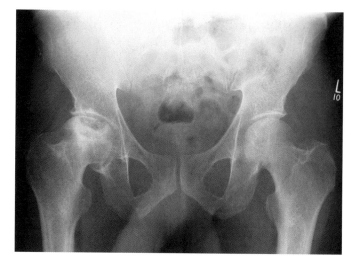

Figure 1.43 Avascular necrosis of the right femoral head due to sickle cell disease

- **Ix** Blood film, Hb electrophoresis
- **Rx** *Supportive*: aggressive analgesia, antibiotics and fluids when needed
- **Cx** Gallstones, leg ulcers, avascular necrosis of femoral head, chronic renal disease

MACROCYTIC ANAEMIA ($\uparrow$ MCV)

MEGALOBLASTIC ANAEMIA

- **A** Vitamin B_{12}/folate deficiency
- **P** Large erythroblasts in the bone marrow – faulty maturation due to defective DNA synthesis

VITAMIN B_{12} DEFICIENCY

- **P** Vitamin B_{12} binds to IF (intrinsic factor) which is produced by the stomach parietal cells, and then is absorbed in the terminal ileum
- **A** Pernicious anaemia deficiency (Ab against gastric parietal cells, IF), malabsorption (secondary to Crohn's disease affecting the terminal ileum, bacterial overgrowth) post-total gastrectomy, dietary
- **Si** Pernicious anaemia can be associated with other autoimmune conditions, neurological manifestations (peripheral neuropathy, subacute combined degeneration of the cord, dementia), infertility
- **Ix** $\uparrow$ MCV, $\downarrow B_{12}$, $\downarrow$ platelets, $\downarrow$ WBC, IF antibodies, Schilling test, folate levels
- **Rx** i.m. B_{12} injections

INFORMATION BOX: SCHILLING TEST

A Schilling test is performed to detect whether the body can absorb B_{12} normally.

A small dose of *radioactive* B_{12} is given orally with a large intramuscular dose of *normal* B_{12}. Urine is then collected to see if the radioactive B_{12} is excreted (and hence has been absorbed).

If negative, then the test can be repeated with the addition of oral IF. If the test becomes positive after this, then the diagnosis is pernicious anaemia (lack of IF). If the test is still negative the diagnosis is small bowel disease.

FOLATE DEFICIENCY

 Folate is normally found in green vegetables, and absorbed in the upper part of the small intestine

 Dietary inadequacy, malabsorption, increased requirements (pregnancy, haemolysis), folate antagonists e.g. methotrexate

(Ix) ↑MCV, ↓folate

(Rx) Folic acid supplements

NON-MEGALOBLASTIC ANAEMIA

 Normoblastic bone marrow
↑MCV

Box 1.28 NON-MEGALOBLASTIC CAUSES OF MACROCYTOSIS

- Alcohol excess (common)
- Reticulocytosis
- Hypothyroidism
- Physiological (pregnancy)
- Liver disease

 Treatment of underlying cause

NORMOCYTIC NORMOCHROMIC ANAEMIA (ANAEMIA OF CHRONIC DISEASE)

 Chronic renal failure, chronic infections, rheumatoid arthritis, connective tissue diseases, malignant diseases

(Ix) → ferritin, ↓serum iron, ↓total iron-binding capacity (TIBC)

(Rx) Treat underlying cause, erythropoietin injections in CRF

APLASTIC ANAEMIA

(A) Due to a decrease in pluripotential stem cells resulting in pancytopenia
Can be idiopathic, congenital or secondary: drugs (e.g. phenytoin, carbamazepine), parvovirus, viral hepatitis; ionizing radiation

(Sy) SOB, palpitations, chest pain, bleeding, easy bruising, recurrent infection

(Ix) FBC, blood film, bone marrow aspirate and trephine, LFT, viral titres

Rx Remove or treat precipitant, supportive (i.e. blood and platelet transfusions; G-CSF (granulocyte cell-stimulating factor)

Specific: immunosuppression, bone marrow transplantation

Px Relates to severity

HAEMOLYSIS

P Abnormal premature destruction of RBCs

Box 1.29 CAUSES OF HAEMOLYSIS

- *Congenital*:
  - hereditary spherocytosis
  - thalassaemia
  - sickle cell disease
  - G6PD (glucose-6-phosphate dehydrogenase) deficiency
- *Acquired*:
  - autoimmune haemolytic anaemia (AIHA)
  - microangiopathic haemolytic anaemia (MAHA)
  - infection

Si Pallor, jaundice, splenomegaly

Ix *Bloods*: ↑ unconjugated bilirubin, ↑ LDH, ↓ haptoglobins, ↑ reticulocyte count, Coombs' test

Blood film: polychromasia

HEREDITARY SPHEROCYTOSIS

A Autosomal dominant

P Defect in cell membrane, results in increased cell fragility

Si Splenomegaly, mild anaemia

Ix *Blood film*: spherocytes (small spherical darkly stained RBCs with no central pallor)

Rx Nil specific unless symptomatic → splenectomy

G6PD DEFICIENCY

A X-linked

P Normally G6PD generates NADPH, which is responsible for maintaining a healthy Hb so that it can withstand the stresses caused by drugs, sepsis

Deficiency of G6PD therefore means that Hb breaks down under stress resulting in haemolytic anaemia

Causes of haemolysis include analgesics, antimalarials and antibiotics

Rx Avoidance of drugs known to precipitate haemolysis

COAGULATION DISORDERS

AUTOIMMUNE THROMBOCYTOPENIC PURPURA (AITP)

P Due to antibodies against the antigens on the platelet surface resulting in removal via the reticuloendothelial system

A Affects middle-aged women and children

(Sy) Recurrent epistaxis, ecchymosis, gingival bleeding, menorrhagia

(Ix) FBC ($\downarrow$ platelets), blood film, bone marrow biopsy

(Rx) Only if platelets $<30 \times 10^9$/L, high dose of glucocorticoids, immunoglobulin infusion; if resistant consider splenectomy

HAEMOPHILIA A AND B

(A) Inherited disorders of coagulation, X-linked recessive (only males suffer from disease, females carry disease)

(P) Haemophilia A: deficiency of Factor VIIIc

Haemophilia B: deficiency of Factor IX

(Sy) Haemarthrosis, secondary arthritis, spontaneous soft tissue bleeds (i.e. psoas, gastrocnemius), GI bleeding, haematuria, loin pain

(Ix) $\uparrow$ APTT, $\rightarrow$ PT, $\rightarrow$ von Willebrand factor (vWF), platelets

Haemophilia A: $\downarrow$ factor VIII

Haemophilia B: $\downarrow$ factor IX

(Rx) *Haemophilia A:* purified factor VIIIc, desmopressin (increases factor VIII levels)

Haemophilia B: factor IX injections

VON WILLEBRAND'S DISEASE

(A) Most common inherited disorder of coagulation

Various subtypes, most common is autosomal dominant

(P) Associated with either low or abnormal vWF

(Sy) Mucosal/capillary bleeding, easy bruising

(Ix) FBC, $\uparrow$ APTT, $\rightarrow$ PT, $\downarrow$ factor VIIIc + vWF and $\uparrow$ bleeding time

(Rx) vWF concentrate, DDAVP (vasopressin) infusions, cryoprecipitate, fresh-frozen plasma (FFP)

DISSEMINATED INTRAVASCULAR COAGULATION (DIC)

(P) Pathological activation of coagulation resulting in bleeding and widespread microvascular thrombosis

---

Box 1.30 CAUSES OF DISSEMINATED INTRAVASCULAR COAGULATION

- *Infection*: Gram −ve, meningococcal, viral
- *Malignancy*: solid tumours, leukaemia
- *Obstetric*: eclampsia, retained placenta, amniotic fluid embolus
- *Immunological*: anaphylaxis
- *Liver disease*: acute liver disease, cirrhosis

(Sy) Haemorrhage, widespread microthrombi, large-vessel thrombosis, haemorrhagic tissue necrosis

(Ix) $\uparrow$ PT, $\uparrow$ APTT, $\uparrow$ thrombin time (TT), $\downarrow$ fibrinogen, $\uparrow$ fibrin degradation products (FDP)

(Rx) Treat underlying condition, FFP, platelets, cryoprecipitate

DEEP VEIN THROMBOSIS (DVT)

(P) Clot that occurs in a deep vein, most commonly in the lower limb

(A) Immobility (including long car/plane journeys), recent major operation/trauma, pregnancy, OCP

Associated with malignancy, pro-coagulant states (see thrombophilia below)

Sy Increased swelling, erythema, warm, tender over site of thrombosis

Ix Duplex USS of the affected limb, D-dimer

Px Anticoagulate, exclude underlying malignancy or possible thrombophilia (see below), TED (thromboembolic deterrent) stockings

Cx Pulmonary embolus, post-thrombotic limb

THROMBOPHILIA

P Conditions which induce a pro-coagulant state resulting in thrombosis, affects 5–7 per cent of the population

---

Box 1.31 CAUSES OF THROMBOPHILIA

- *Primary*:
  - protein C deficiency
  - protein S deficiency
  - antithrombin III deficiency
  - factor V Leiden
  - homocystinuria

- *Secondary*:
  - malignancy
  - immobility
  - major surgery (especially orthopaedic)
  - OCP
  - smoking
  - pregnancy
  - antiphospholipid syndrome

Sy Relate to the location of the clot

PE: SOB, haemoptysis, pleuritic chest pain

DVT: calf swelling, pain, tenderness, erythema

Ix Patients should be investigated if:
- thromboembolism <45 years, or family history
- recurrent thromboembolism/miscarriage
- thrombosis at an unusual site

FBC (exclude polycythaemia, myelofibrosis), APTT, PT, fibrinogen, blood film

Rx Anticoagulation, avoid precipitants e.g. OCP

PREMALIGNANT DISORDERS

POLYCYTHAEMIA

P ↑RCC, ↑PCV (haematocrit), ↑Hb

A ♂ > ♀, mean age 50–60 years

Primary, due to a clonal stem cell disorder (polycythaemia rubra vera), or secondary (due to either hypoxia → high altitude, pulmonary disease or inappropriate erythropoietin secretion → cerebellar haemangioblastoma, renal tumour)

Sy Headaches, dizziness, pruritus after bathing, loss of consciousness, gout

Si Facial plethora, bleeding, splenomegaly, bruising

Ix FBC, nuclear medicine red cell mass, abdominal USS

Rx If primary: venesection, antiplatelet drugs for digital microvascular occlusion and TIA; if secondary treat underlying cause

Cx Transformation to myelofibrosis/acute myelogenous leukaemia (AML)

MYELOFIBROSIS

P Clonal proliferation of haemopoietic stem cells leading to bone marrow fibrosis

A Mean age 60 years

Si Pallor, bruising, oral thrush, massive splenomegaly, systemic symptoms

Ix FBC, blood film (leucoerythroblastic + tear-drop RBC), bone marrow trephine biopsy

Rx *Supportive:* blood transfusion
Specific: hydroxycarbamide, splenectomy, thalidomide

Cx DIC, transformation to AML, liver failure

Px Poor prognostic factors: ↑ age, anaemia, leucopenia, abnormal marrow karyotype

MYELODYSPLASIA

P Clonal disorder of bone marrow, produces morphological and functionally abnormal blood cells

Sy Features of anaemia, bacterial infections, bleeding

Ix FBC (↑ MCV, ↓ Hb, neutrophils, platelets); blood film, bone marrow biopsy

Rx *Supportive:* blood, platelet transfusions, antibiotics
Specific: treatment limited, in young patients allogeneic bone marrow transplantation may be curative

Px Poor, after 2–3 years one-third transform to AML
Median survival 3 years

MALIGNANCIES

ACUTE LYMPHOBLASTIC LEUKAEMIA

P Haematological malignancy resulting in ↑ production of lymphoblasts

A Commoner in children, peak age 4 years, bimodal in adults 15–25 years or >75 years

Sy Bleeding (bruising, menorrhagia, epistaxis), lethargy, SOB, arthralgia, malaise, recurrent infection, CNS infiltration, testicular disease

Ix FBC, clotting, blood film, cytochemistry, immunophenotyping, cytogenetics

Rx *Supportive:* treat infections, bleeding
Specific: chemotherapy, bone marrow transplant

Px Childhood good, adults poor

Cx Haemorrhage, thrombosis, tumour lysis syndrome (hyperuricaemia and renal failure) secondary to treatment

ACUTE MYELOGENOUS LEUKAEMIA

P Haematological malignancy resulting in the overproduction of immature myeloid WBCs

A Peak age of onset 70 years, rare under 20 years
Risk of transformation from chronic myeloid leukaemia (CML), myelodysplasia, myelofibrosis, polycythaemia rubra vera (PRV)

Sy Malaise, lethargy, anaemia, bleeding, recurrent infections

Si Purpura, organomegaly, lymphadenopathy, splenomegaly. DIC associated with M3 subtype.

Ix FBC (↓ Hb, normal platelets), blood film, bone marrow trephine (Auer cells), lymph node biopsy, abdominal USS

Rx *Supportive:* blood transfusions, antibiotics
Specific: chemotherapy

Px Long-term survival 50 per cent

Cx Relapse of the disease, severe bleeding and infection, CNS infiltration

CHRONIC LYMPHOCYTIC LEUKAEMIA

P Monoclonal malignancy resulting in functionally incompetent lymphocytes

A Occurs in those aged over 60 years

Sy Recurrent infections, bleeding, anorexia, sweating, malaise, abdominal discomfort, malaise

Si Lymphadenopathy, splenomegaly, hepatomegaly, petechiae, pallor

Ix FBC (lymphocytosis, anaemia, thrombocytopenia), blood film (smudge cells), hypogammaglobulinaemia, bone marrow biopsy, lymph node biopsy

Rx *Supportive:* blood transfusions, antibiotics
Specific: chlorambucil ± prednisolone, splenectomy

Cx Increased risk of second malignancy, autoimmune haemolytic anaemia, idiopathic thrombocytopenic purpura (ITP)

CHRONIC MYELOID LEUKAEMIA

P Malignancy of granulocytes leads to ↑ production of myeloid precursors, with their differentiation ability still intact
Associated with the Philadelphia chromosome (translocation between 9 and 22 resulting in the *bcr-abl* gene that produces tyrosine kinase)

A Occurs in middle-aged and elderly

Sy Anaemia, weight loss, lassitude, anorexia, sweating, gout, bleeding, priapism, low-grade fever

Si Bruising, petechiae, splenomegaly, hepatomegaly

Ix FBC (↑ WBC), clotting, blood film, cytochemistry, immunophenotyping, cytogenetics

Rx *Supportive*: blood transfusions, antibiotics
Specific: alkylating agents, splenectomy, allogeneic bone marrow transplantation

HODGKIN'S LYMPHOMA

P Malignancy of the lymphatic system, involves clonal expansion of B and T white blood cells
Binucleate Reed–Sternberg cells ('owl's eye') are characteristic of Hodgkin's lymphoma

A Rare: <1500 new cases per annum in UK
Bimodal age distribution: peaks at 20–35 years and 50–60 years

S Painless lymphadenopathy – localized or generalized. Cervical chain is commonest site
Constitutional or 'B' symptoms are experienced in up to a quarter of patients: these include fever, weight loss (>10 per cent), pruritus, sweats

Ix *Bloods*: FBC, U&E, LFTs, LDH, ESR
Imaging: CXR, CT scan of the chest/abdomen/pelvis
Histology:
– Biopsy of lymph node
– Bone marrow aspirate and trephine

Box 1.32 ANN ARBOR STAGING SYSTEM FOR HODGKIN'S LYMPHOMA

- *Stage I*: confined to single lymph node group
- *Stage II*: two or more lymph node groups but confined to one side of the diaphragm
- *Stage III*: as for Stage II but both sides of diaphragm
- *Stage IV*: involvement of extralymphatic sites e.g. bone marrow

Staging includes absence (A) or presence (B) of systemic symptoms

---

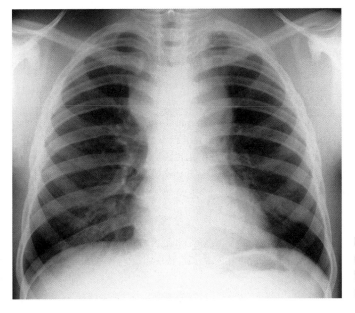

Figure 1.44 Anterior mediastinal mass due to lymphadenopathy from Hodgkin's lymphoma

Rx Localized disease (Stage IA and IIA): radiotherapy to involved and adjacent lymph node
Extensive disease (Stage III and IV): chemotherapy
If B symptoms are present: chemotherapy

Px 10-year survival rates vary from ~50 per cent for Stage IV to 80 per cent for Stage IA disease

NON-HODGKIN'S LYMPHOMA (NHL)

A $10 \times$ more common than Hodgkin's lymphoma
Increases with age and slight male preponderance
Geographical variation: Burkitt's lymphoma common in Africa
Viruses are implicated e.g. EBV, herpes simplex virus (HSV)
Immunosuppression is also a risk factor (including HIV/AIDS)

(P) B-cell lymphoma (90 per cent of cases)
T-cell lymphoma (10 per cent of cases)
NHL can be classified as low, intermediate and high grade
(S) Lymphadenopathy (60–70 per cent), hepatosplenomegaly, 'B' symptoms (as above)
(Ix) As for Hodgkin's lymphoma
Staging: as for Hodgkin's lymphoma
Most patients present in Stage III or IV
(Rx) *Stage I and II*: radiotherapy to the involved and adjacent lymph node or chemotherapy (depending on predominant cell subtype)
Stage III and IV: chemotherapy and interferon
Intermediate and high grade: high-dose chemotherapy
Consider autologous bone marrow transplantation in unresponsive or recurrent disease
(Px) 10-year survival rates vary from ~35 per cent for Stage IV to 80 per cent for Stage I disease

MULTIPLE MYELOMA

(P) Malignancy of plasma cells resulting in abnormal plasma cells: ↑monoclonal antibodies
(A) Peak age of incidence 60 years
(Sy) Musculoskeletal (bone pain, pathological fractures, vertebral collapse, kyphosis), spinal cord compression, respiratory infections, anaemia (SOB, palpitations, lethargy), headaches + somnolence (due to ↑viscosity)
(Si) Bleeding, bruising, purpura, pallor, bony tenderness
(Ix) *Bloods*: FBC, blood film (leucoerythroblastic, rouleaux), bone marrow biopsy, ↑Ca^{2+}, ↑urea + creatinine, protein electrophoresis (shows monoclonal band), ↑↑ESR
Urine: Bence–Jones protein (immunoglobulin light chains in urine, not picked up on dipstick)
X-ray: skeletal survey looking for lytic lesions
(Rx) Analgesia, radiotherapy to bony lesions, bisphosphonates, steroids, chemotherapy, plasmapheresis, thalidomide, bone marrow transplantation
(Cx) Amyloidosis, renal failure, spinal cord compression, bone fractures
(Px) Median survival 3 years

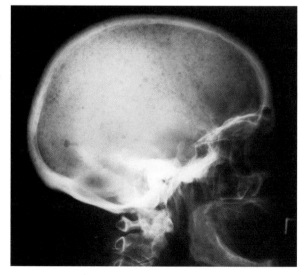

Figure 1.45 Widespread small lytic lesions in the cranial vault from multiple myeloma

INFECTIOUS DISEASES

AIDS (ACQUIRED IMMUNE DEFICIENCY SYNDROME)

(P) HIV (human immunodeficiency virus) infects CD4+ cells (T-helper cells) and destroys them; viral RNA is converted into DNA by **reverse transcriptase**; as the cell replicates protein it also replicates the HIV
When a patient's CD4 count is < 200 cells/mm^3 the patient is said to have AIDS

(A) Transmitted by body secretions: intravenous drug use, sexual intercourse, vertical transmission, blood transfusions, tattoos

(S) Often there is a flu-like illness at the time of seroconversion; usually the first symptoms are due to opportunistic infections; common symptoms include fever, weight loss, lymphadenopathy, weakness

(Ix) HIV test, CD4 count, viral load

(Rx) *HAART (highly active anti-retroviral treatment)*
  – Nucleoside reverse transcriptase inhibitors (NRTI)
  – Non-nucleoside reverse transcriptase inhibitors (NNRTI)
  – Protease inhibitors
New drugs: entry inhibitors, integrase inhibitors, assembly inhibitors, immunotherapy

(Cx) Drug resistance, opportunistic infections (see below), death

OPPORTUNISTIC INFECTIONS (OI)

(P) Infections which do not normally cause problems in a fully functioning immune system can cause fatal disease in AIDS. OIs occur when the CD4 count <200 cells/mm^3
There are multiple OIs, each which can present in different ways. Examples are shown in Box 1.33.

Box 1.33 DISEASES CAUSED BY OPPORTUNISTIC INFECTIONS

- *Fungal*: candidiasis, coccidioidomycosis, aspergillosis, cryptococcal meningitis
- *Bacterial*: *Mycobacterium avium* complex, tuberculosis
- *Protozoa*: *Pneumocystis carinii* pneumonia (PCP), cryptosporidiosis, toxoplasmosis
- *Viral*: CMV, HSV, human papilloma virus (HPV), herpes zoster virus (HZV), oral hairy leucoplakia, progressive multifocal leucoencephalopathy
- *Malignancy*: lymphoma (EBV), Kaposi's sarcoma (human herpesvirus-8), anal/cervical cancer (HPV)
- *Neurological*: AIDS dementia, peripheral neuropathy

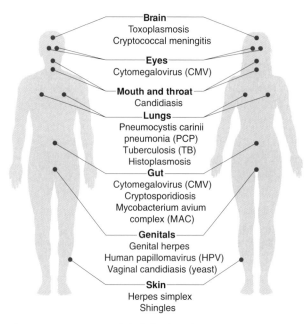

Figure 1.46 Opportunistic infections in AIDS

METHICILLIN-RESISTANT *STAPHYLOCOCCUS AUREUS* (MRSA)

P MRSA is commonly found on the skin or in the nose. Methicillin is the laboratory equivalent of flucloxacillin

A Usually occurs in hospitalized patients, at risk of cross-infection

S Dependent on the site of infection; it can range from asymptomatic colonization to bacteraemia

Ix Wound swabs

Rx Antibiotics (vancomycin/teicoplanin), isolation and barrier nursing to prevent cross-infection

VANCOMYCIN-RESISTANT ENTEROCOCCUS (VRE)

P Enterococci are part of the intestinal flora; spread by direct contact with the faeces of an infected patient; usually due to poor hygiene

A Hospitalized patients, chronic disease, immunosuppressed, previous antibiotic use

S Dependent on the site of infection: urinary tract infection (UTI), wound infections, endocarditis, bacteraemia, intra-abdominal infections

Ix FBC, septic screen

Rx Isolation and barrier nursing; combination of antibiotics is required – discuss with microbiologist as per regime

CLOSTRIDIUM DIFFICILE TOXIN

P *Clostridium difficile* is a Gram-positive anaerobe; it can colonize the colon and produce two toxins: A (enterotoxin) and B (cytotoxin)

A Antibiotic use, hospital stay, increased risk with older age

S Diarrhoea, fever, abdominal pain

Ix Stool MC&S, FBC ($\uparrow$ WCC)

Rx Vancomycin, metronidazole, isolation and barrier nursing
Cx Pseudomembranous colitis, toxic megacolon, sepsis

BOTULISM

P *Clostridium botulinum* produces heat-resistant spores causing neuromuscular blockade
A Canned foods, inadequate cooking
Si Nausea, diarrhoea and vomiting, visual disturbance, paralysis
Ix Faecal analysis for toxin
Px Poor, >50 per cent mortality

INFECTIOUS MONONUCLEOSIS

P Caused by Epstein–Barr virus (EBV)
A EBV is spread by salivary secretions; has also been transmitted by blood transfusion and bone marrow transplant
Sy Fatigue, malaise, fever, myalgia
Si Papular rash, pharyngitis, lymphadenopathy, splenomegaly
Ix ↑WCC (lymphocytosis), ↓ platelets, ↑LFT, monospot, Paul Bunnell test, EBV titres
Rx Usually self-limiting and treatment is supportive;
Cx Bacterial superinfection, haemolytic anaemia, splenic rupture, myocarditis, pericarditis, meningitis, encephalitis, Guillain–Barré syndrome
EBV has also been associated with Burkitt's lymphoma, nasopharyngeal carcinoma, Hodgkin's disease and lymphoproliferative disease in immunosuppressed patients

HERPES SIMPLEX VIRUS (HSV)

P Double-stranded DNA virus, causes wide variety of syndromes
A Transmission via infected saliva, genital contact
Sy Cold sores (usually HSV-1), genital herpes (HSV-1 and -2)
Si Pyrexia, herpetic vesicles, cervicitis, urethritis
Ix Viral culture
Rx Aciclovir: topical for cold sores, systemic for genital herpes

CHICKENPOX

P Varicella zoster infection
A Usually affects children, person-to-person spread
S Fever, headache, vesicular rash
Ix Clinical, viral culture
Rx Supportive, aciclovir if immunocompromised or pregnant
Cx Pneumonia, shingles, birth defects if pregnant

MUMPS

P Parotitis as a result of infection with a paramyxovirus
A Droplet/direct contact transmission
Can be prevented by vaccination with MMR (measles mumps and rubella) vaccine
S Pyrexia, headache, parotid swelling
Ix Clinical diagnosis
Rx Supportive

Cx Epididymo-orchitis, subfertility, meningitis, pancreatitis

MEASLES

P Paramyxovirus infection

A Droplet spread

Can be prevented by vaccination with MMR

S Pyrexia, Koplik spots (small grey lesions on buccal mucosa), maculopapular rash

Ix Clinical

Rx Supportive, analgesia

Cx Common: pneumonia, gastroenteritis, subacute sclerosing panencephalitis (reactivation of virus in brain ~10 years after infection: almost universally fatal)

MALARIA

P Transmitted by mosquito bites; four *Plasmodium* species: *falciparum, vivax, ovale,* and *malariae*; *vivax* and *ovale* species can remain dormant as hypnozoites and cause recurrent infections

A Occurs in tropical areas

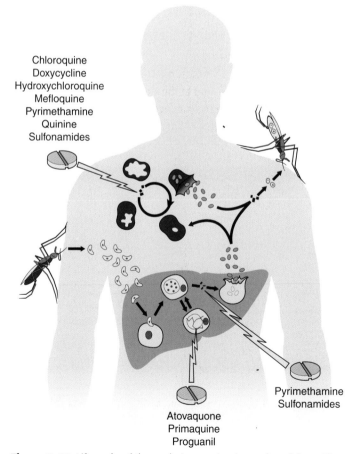

Figure 1.47 Life cycle of the malaria parasite (reproduced from Simonsen T, Aarbakke J, Kay I, Coleman I, Sinnot P and Lysaa R, *Illustrated Pharmacology For Nurses*, London: Hodder Arnold, 2006 with kind permission by the illustrator Roy A Lysaa)

Sy Fever, fatigue, myalgia, headache, nausea, vomiting
Si Tachycardia, anaemia, jaundice, splenomegaly,
Ix Blood smears, FBC (anaemia), ↑ESR, ↑CRP, U&E, LFT
Rx Quinine, mefloquine, doxycycline, chloroquine
Cx Falciparum malaria: cerebral malaria, hypoglycaemia, renal impairment

TYPHOID

P Infection with *Salmonella typhi*
A Faecal–oral transmission via contaminated food or water
Preventable by vaccination
S Fever, headache, diarrhoea, rose spots (blanching maculopapular rash on trunk), splenomegaly
Ix Blood, urine, stool cultures, serology
Rx Ciprofloxacin (increasing resistance worldwide), fluids
Cx Pneumonia, haemolysis, meningitis, death

SEXUALLY TRANSMITTED INFECTIONS

SYPHILIS

P Caused by a spirochaete, *Treponema pallidum*
A Sexually transmitted infection
S *Primary syphilis*: primary lesion is the **chancre**, a raised painless papule with an ulcerated centre, usually found at the site of inoculation; lymphadenopathy
Secondary syphilis: widespread mucocutaneous lesions, fever, malaise, headache, lymphadenopathy, sore throat; other systems rarely involved
Tertiary syphilis: characterized by the **gumma**, usually found in the liver, bone and testes
 Microscopy of fluid from mucocutaneous lesions, VDRL (venereal diseases research laboratory), *Treponema pallidum* haemagglutination assay (TPHA)
Other investigations to assess for complications include CXR, CT/MRI, lumbar puncture
Rx Penicillin
 Congenital syphilis: spontaneous abortion, birth defects
Cardiovascular syphilis: aortic aneurysm, aortic regurgitation
Neurosyphilis: tabes dorsalis, brain atrophy, Argyll Robertson pupil

GONORRHOEA

P Bacterial infection caused by *Neisseria gonorrhoeae*
A Sexually transmitted infection
Sy Purulent penile discharge, often asymptomatic in women
Ix Microscopy of discharge reveals characteristic Gram-negative diplococci
Rx Cephalosporin, widespread antibiotic resistance
Cx Septic arthritis, most common cause of monoarthritis in sexually active adults

CHLAMYDIA

(P) Causative organism *Chlamydia trachomatis*
(A) Most common sexually transmitted infection in UK
(S) ♀ usually none, sometimes cervicitis/cystitis, lower abdominal pain, intermenstrual bleeding
♂ often asymptomatic, discharge, dysuria
(Ix) Urine testing for *Chlamydia*
(Rx) Azithromycin, widespread resistance
(Cx) Peri-hepatitis (Fitz-Hugh–Curtis syndrome)

GENITAL WARTS

(P) Infection with HPV causes warts
(A) Skin-to-skin contact during sexual contact
(Sy) Soft, fleshy warts anywhere in genital area
(Ix) Clinical
(Rx) No known cure, topical treatment with liquid nitrogen, podophyllin
(Cx) Implicated in pathogenesis of cervical cancer and anal cancer

DERMATOLOGY

DERMATOLOGICAL TERMS

- **Abscess:** a local accumulation of pus
- **Atrophy:** wasting away/diminution
- **Bulla:** blister >5 cm
- **Comedone:** plug of sebaceous and dead skin material stuck in the opening of a hair follicle: open (blackhead) or closed (whitehead)
- **Erosion:** loss of epithelium
- **Erythema:** redness of the skin
- **Hyperpigmentation:** increased pigmentation
- **Hypopigmentation:** decreased pigmentation
- **Macule:** a small, flat, distinct, coloured area of skin <10 mm in diameter
- **Nodule:** raised lesion >1 cm (an enlargement of a papule)
- **Papule:** small, circumscribed, palpable lesion
- **Plaque:** large elevated solid lesions
- **Purpura:** non-blanching, haemorrhagic lesions, >3 mm
- **Pustule:** blister containing pus
- **Scaling:** an increase in the dead cells on the surface of the skin (stratum corneum)
- **Telangiectasia:** prominent cutaneous dilated blood vessels
- **Ulcer:** full-thickness loss of epidermis or epithelium, may be covered with a dark-coloured crust (eschar)
- **Vesicle:** small, fluid-filled blister
- **Wheals:** cutaneous oedema due to leaking capillaries

ECZEMA

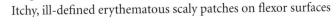

P *Atopic eczema*: begins in infancy. Occurs in 5 per cent of those <5 years old; 25 per cent of patients have a first-degree relative with atopy (an inherited altered immune reactivity i.e. asthma, hay fever, conjunctivitis or eczema)

Exogenous eczema: irritant contact dermatitis, allergic contact dermatitis

Sy Itchy, ill-defined erythematous scaly patches on flexor surfaces

Si Erythematous scaly patches, oedema, vesicles

Ix Clinical diagnosis, can be associated with elevated IgE

Patch testing for contact dermatitis

Rx Atopic eczema:
- *topical*: emollients, tar, steroids, psoralen plus ultraviolet A (PUVA)
- *systemic*: oral antihistamines, antibiotics for infections, immunosuppressants (azathioprine)

Avoid irritants, if patients develop eczema herpeticum i.e. secondary infection with HSV then the patient needs to be admitted for i.v. aciclovir

Px Atopic eczema: 40 per cent resolve after 5 years, 90 per cent between 15 and 20 years

PSORIASIS

A Polygenic susceptibility

Arthropathy is associated with HLA B27

Exacerbating factors include drugs (antimalarials, β-blockers, alcohol, lithium), stress and infections e.g. streptococcal sore throat can precipitate guttate psoriasis

(P) Several subtypes exist including stable chronic plaque, guttate, erythrodermic, and pustular psoriasis

(Si) Salmon-coloured silver scaly lesions often involving the scalp, behind the ear, predominantly on extensor surfaces but can occur anywhere

Lesions can be plaques, nummular (coin-shaped) or guttate (raindrop-shaped)

Exhibits the Koebner phenomenon (lesions occur over sites of trauma)

Nail signs: nail pitting, onycholysis, nail dystrophy, subungual hyperkeratosis

(Ix) Clinical diagnosis, but can do a biopsy

(Rx) *Supportive*: emollients

Topical: tar, topical steroids, dithranol, ultraviolet B (UVB), PUVA

Systemic: PUVA, methotrexate, ciclosporin, hydroxycarbamide, sulfasalazine

(Px) Only 1 per cent of patients with psoriasis develop psoriatic arthropathy

LICHEN PLANUS

(Si) *Skin*: pruritic eruption of violaceous, shiny, polygonal papules with Wickham's striae (characteristic white lines)

Mouth: oral involvement (white or grey streaks forming a linear or reticular pattern on a violaceous background)

Nails: onycholysis, dystrophy, longitudinal ridging, pterygium (scarring of the nail bed)

Scalp: alopecia

(Rx) Self-limiting, resolves within 8–12 months

URTICARIA

(A) Wide variety of causes (see Box 1.34)

Box 1.34 CAUSES OF URTICARIA

- *Recent illness*
- *Drugs*: ACE inhibitors, anaesthetics, antibiotics
- *Infection*: amoebiasis, malaria
- *Foods*: shellfish, fish, eggs, cheese, chocolate, nuts, berries, tomatoes
- *Synthetic products*: perfumes, creams, nail polish, nickel, rubber, latex, industrial chemicals, detergents
- *Pets*: exposure to new animals (dander)
- *Pregnancy*: usually occurs in last trimester and typically resolves spontaneously soon after delivery
- *Environmental*: dust, mould, chemicals, or plants
- *Idiopathic*

(Si) Itchy blanching red wheals (circumscribed areas of raised erythema and oedema of the superficial dermis) in response to a precipitant

Acute form of urticaria lasts <4–6 weeks, and the chronic form lasts >4–6 weeks

(Ix) *Bloods*: ANA titres, hepatitis B + C, TFT

(Rx) Identify underlying cause, remove the precipitant and give symptomatic relief (antihistamines, steroids)

PEMPHIGUS

(A) Rare, most common at 45–50 years

(P) Direct action of an antibody attack on the intra-epidermal desmosomal structure

(Sy) Bullous lesions/blisters which may be confined to mucous membranes, but can occur on trunk, scalp and other parts of the body; the blisters rupture easily as they are intra-epithelial

(Ix) *Biopsy*: intra-epidermal blister with acantholysis

Immunology: direct immunofluorescence intercellular IgG and C3

(Rx) *Local*: wet dressings, lotions

Systemic: high-dose steroids, immunosuppressants, i.v. fluids

(Px) Prior to steroids, poor prognosis

(Cx) Secondary infection, sepsis, extensive loss of body fluids and electrolytes

PEMPHIGOID

(P) Autoimmune reaction against the basement membrane

(A) Most common in the elderly

(Si) Initially patients develop erythematous and eczematous areas on the trunk and limb, which then develop tense blisters; can be pruritic, rarely affects the mucosal membranes, bullae usually heal without scarring

(Ix) *Biopsy*: positive direct immunofluorescence demonstrating IgG and C3 at the basement membrane

(Rx) Steroids, azathioprine can be used as a steroid-sparing agent

ACNE VULGARIS

(A) Common skin disease that affects 85–100 per cent of people at some time during their lives

(Si) Characterized by non-inflammatory follicular papules or comedones, in severe cases inflammatory papules, pustules, and nodules

Affects the areas of skin with the densest population of sebaceous follicles; include the face, the upper part of the chest, and the back

(Rx) *Topical*: retinoids, antibiotics

Systemic: antibiotics (tetracyclines), OCP, isotretinoin

PITYRIASIS ROSEA

(Sy) May be prodromal symptoms prior to the development of the rash

(Si) Papular skin eruption that begins as a herald patch (pink oval patch 3–6 cm in diameter), normally initially found on the back before becoming distributed in a Christmas tree pattern

(Ix) Exclude treponemal infection

(Rx) Normally self-limiting, in very severe cases topical steroids

INFECTIONS

TINEA (DERMATOPHYTOSIS, RINGWORM)

(P) Dermatophytes are a group of fungi (ringworm) that invade the dead keratin of skin, hair, and nails.

Box 1.35 SUBTYPES OF TINEA INFESTATION

- *Tinea capitis*: scalp hair
- *Tinea corporis*: trunk and extremities
- *Tinea manuum*: palms
- *Tinea pedis*: soles, and interdigital webs
- *Tinea cruris*: groin
- *Tinea barbae*: beard area and neck
- *Tinea faciale*: face
- *Tinea unguium* (onychomycosis): nail

(Si) Pruritic lesions, classical lesion: central clearing surrounded by an advancing, red, scaly, elevated border. One or more lesions may appear, commonly in the groin, feet and axillae.
Nails: onychomycosis
(Ix) Microscopy of scrapings
(Rx) Topical imidazole, systemic terbinafine
(Px) Infection resolves within 1–2/52 with treatment (longer for onychomycosis)
(Cx) Secondary infection

PITYRIASIS VERSICOLOR
(P) Caused by yeasts of *Pityrosporum orbiculare* (can also be normal commensal)
(A) Occurs in hot, humid countries, or patients who sweat a lot
(Si) Flaky discoloured patches appear mainly on the chest and back, trunk and arms; the patches may be pink, coppery brown or paler than surrounding skin; mildly itchy
(Ix) Wood's light: yellow, green fluorescence, microscopy of scrapings
(Rx) Topical and systemic antifungal agents used

CELLULITIS
(P) Superficial skin infection due to either staphylococcal or streptococcal subgroups
(A) Predisposed by trauma, oedema or tinea pedis
(Si) Painful, swelling, warmth and erythema over affected site, pyrexia
(Ix) FBC, blood cultures, swabs over affected area
(Rx) Antibiotics (penicillin and flucloxacillin)
(Cx) Sepsis

SCABIES
(P) Infestation of the skin with the microscopic mite *Sarcoptes scabiei*; very contagious
May take up to 4–6 weeks before symptoms occur
(Sy) Severe itchiness
(Si) Symmetrical rash affecting fingers, backs of hands, axillae, breasts and buttock
Excoriated papules and nodules; occasionally burrows are seen
(Ix) Skin scraping: under microscope can see burrow contents
(Rx) Topical insecticides (e.g. permethrin, malathion), imperative to also treat partners and cohabitants

CUTANEOUS MANIFESTATIONS OF SYSTEMIC DISEASE

DERMATITIS HERPETIFORMIS

(P) Strong association with HLA B8, DR3, DQw2 haplotype

(A) Associated with gluten-sensitive enteropathy (coeliac disease)

(Sy) Itchy small blisters on extensor surfaces, buttocks or face

(Ix) *Histology*: subepidermal blisters and microabscesses in the dermal papillae
Immunology: direct immunofluorescence IgA in the papillary tips

(Rx) Dapsone, gluten-free diet

ERYTHEMA NODOSUM

(Si) Tender, erythematous nodules which resolve after 6/52, occur on shins and not associated with scarring

(Rx) Treat underlying cause, supportive treatment of skin lesions

---

Box 1.36 CAUSES OF ERYTHEMA NODOSUM

- Infection: *Streptococcus*, tuberculosis
- Sarcoidosis
- Inflammatory bowel disease: Crohn's disease, ulcerative colitis
- Drugs e.g. sulfonamides, OCP
- Idiopathic

ERYTHEMA MULTIFORME

(Si) Symmetrical eruption of raised target lesions, may be associated with pyrexia
If associated with mucosal involvement known as Stevens–Johnson syndrome

---

Box 1.37 CAUSES OF ERYTHEMA MULTIFORME

- Infection: herpes simplex, *Mycoplasma*, psittacosis, hepatitis B, EBV, histoplasmosis
- Lupus
- Drugs e.g. sulfonamides, antibiotics
- Malignancy including leukaemia
- Pregnancy
- Pre-menstrual
- Sarcoid

(Rx) Steroids, symptomatic treatment

PYODERMA GANGRENOSUM

(A) Inflammatory bowel disease, seronegative rheumatoid arthritis, myeloma

(Si) Painful, rapidly growing ulcerated nodules

(Rx) Oral steroids

(Px) Heals with scarring

LUPUS PERNIO

P Cutaneous manifestation characteristic of chronic sarcoidosis

Si Chronic, indurated violaceous papules or plaques that affect the mid-face, particularly the alar rim of the nose

LUPUS VULGARIS

P Cutaneous tuberculosis affecting the face

Si Brownish tubercles that often heal slowly and leave scars. The lesion spreads with a hyperpigmented margin and a hypopigmented core, often with ulceration

ACANTHOSIS NIGRICANS

A Associated with numerous conditions including malignancy, acromegaly, dermatomyositis, scleroderma and Wilson's disease

Si Lesions begin as hyperpigmented macules/papules and progress on to velvety plaques with associated skin tags. Most commonly occur in axilla, groin and posterior neck

Ix Need to exclude a possible underlying malignancy, diabetes and insulin resistance

Rx None

THROMBOPHLEBITIS MIGRANS

A Associated with stomach and other intra-abdominal malignancies

Si Occurrence of inflammation and thrombosis of veins occurring sequentially at multiple sites

NECROBIOSIS LIPOIDICA

A Associated with diabetes

Si Asymptomatic shiny patches that slowly enlarge over months to years, patches are initially red–brown and progress to yellow, depressed atrophic plaques; most commonly occurs over pre-tibial areas; Koebner phenomenon (i.e. occurs at site of trauma)

Rx Limited but topical and intra-lesion steroids may slow progression

GRANULOMA ANNULARE

A Associated with trauma, diabetes

Si Erythematous, firm, ring-shaped lesions with an elevated edge (diameter 1–5 mm)

Rx Usually self-limiting but can use topical steroids

XANTHELASMA

A Frequently occur in patients with Type II + IV hyperlipidaemia

Si Yellow plaques that occur most commonly near the inner canthus of the eyelid

Rx Control of hypercholesterolaemia

CHAPTER 2

Surgery

Gareth Jones and Simon Phillips

GENERAL SURGERY

SALIVARY GLANDS

INFLAMMATION AND CALCULI

P Inflammation of one or more of the paired salivary glands – parotid, submandibular and sublingual

A Calculi (causing obstruction) or infection (bacterial or mumps)

Sy Lumps, pain and swelling – exacerbated by eating when due to calculus

Si External swellings, erythema ± purulent discharge from duct openings in mouth, bimanual palpation of calculi, lymph node enlargement

Ix X-ray or sialogram (contrast injected into duct) to reveal calculi

Rx *Calculi:* removed via mouth if distal, or gland excision

Bacterial infection: hydration and antibiotics

Mumps: rest and antipyretics

MALIGNANCY

A 80 per cent of tumours involve the parotid gland

P Benign (80 per cent pleomorphic adenoma) or malignant (commonly adenocarcinoma)

Sy Salivary gland lump, pain

Si Palpable swelling, may have evidence of facial nerve (VII) involvement (as nerve VII passes through the parotid)

Ix Sialogram (injection of contrast into salivary duct), computed tomography (CT) or magnetic resonance imaging (MRI)

Rx *Benign*: wide excision of tumour with preservation of facial nerve
Malignant: radical parotidectomy (including facial nerve) and radiotherapy ± lymph node dissection

Cx Post-operative: facial nerve injury, Frey syndrome (facial sweating while eating due to abnormal connection between autonomic and facial nerve fibres)

Px Poor prognosis in malignant tumours (5-year survival ~50 per cent)

OESOPHAGUS

GASTRO-OESOPHAGEAL REFLUX DISEASE (GORD)

Please refer to section in Chapter 1 (p. 35)

PERFORATION

This is a **surgical emergency**

A Oesophagogastroduodenoscopy (OGD) (increased risk if dilatation or biopsy performed), foreign body, external trauma, post-emesis (Boerhaave's syndrome), carcinoma

Sy Chest pain, dysphagia

Si Pyrexia, tachycardia, hypotension, supraclavicular surgical emphysema (air in tissues – produces a 'crackling' sensation on palpation and is visible on X-ray). Signs of systemic sepsis will rapidly develop if undiagnosed

Ix Chest X-ray (CXR): mediastinal surgical emphysema, air/fluid level in pleural cavity. Water-soluble contrast swallow (e.g. Gastrografin)

Rx Small perforation may be managed conservatively: nil by mouth (NBM), i.v. (intravenous) fluids, antibiotics
Larger perforations require urgent surgical repair

Px If operation (when indicated) is delayed >48 h, mortality is >50 per cent

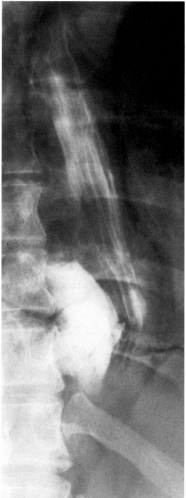

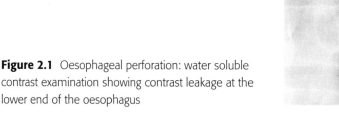

Figure 2.1 Oesophageal perforation: water soluble contrast examination showing contrast leakage at the lower end of the oesophagus

STRICTURES

P Narrowing of any tubular structure e.g. oesophagus

A *Benign*: ingestion of corrosives, GORD, trauma (e.g. OGD), foreign body
Malignant: See p. 110

Sy Dysphagia (initially food > fluid)

Si May be malnourished/cachectic

Ix OGD, barium swallow

Rx Endoscopic dilatation (if unsuccessful or frequently required, may consider surgical resection of stricture)

HIATUS HERNIA

P Herniation of the gastro-oesophageal junction (GOJ) and/or proximal part of stomach through diaphragm into the thorax
Three types:
- sliding (80 per cent): GOJ enters thorax (disturbs cardio-oesophageal sphincter mechanism)
- rolling (5 per cent): proximal part of stomach herniates into thorax
- mixed (15 per cent): combination of rolling and sliding

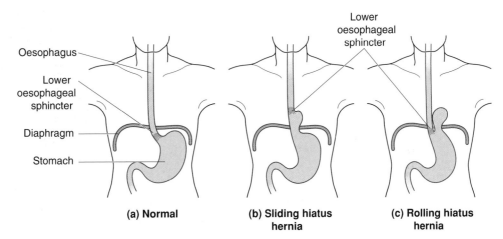

Figure 2.2 Hiatus hernia. (a) Normal oesophagus and stomach; (b) sliding hiatus hernia; (c) rolling/para-oesophageal hiatus hernia

A Classically obese, >50 years, women

Sy Asymptomatic, GORD (in sliding variety)

Ix OGD to assess oesophagitis, barium swallow

Rx *Conservative* : ↓ weight, lifestyle changes as per GORD
Surgical : Nissen's fundoplication (wrap fundus of stomach around lower oesophagus). Indicated in rolling hiatus hernias due to risk of volvulus, and when symptoms/sequelae of GORD are not controlled conservatively

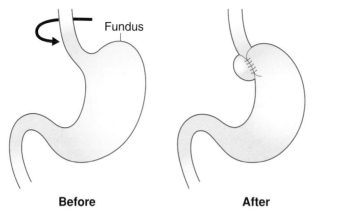

Figure 2.3 Nissen fundoplication

Before   After

MALIGNANCY

 Incidence : ↑ China, ↑↑ Iran versus UK

Associated with smoking, alcohol, diet, Barrett's oesophagus, achalasia

(P) Upper two-thirds squamous carcinoma, lower one-third adenocarcinoma (Barrett's oesophagus associated)

Site: 20 per cent upper one-third, 50 per cent middle one-third, 30 per cent lower one-third (increasing due to Barrett's oesophagus)

(Sy) Progressive dysphagia, general symptoms of malignant disease (i.e. weight loss, anaemia etc.)

(Si) Hoarse voice indicating possible invasion of recurrent laryngeal nerve

(Ix) CXR, barium swallow, OGD + biopsy/brushings, CT to stage

(Rx) An attempt at curative oesophagectomy (e.g. Ivor–Lewis) is appropriate in <50 per cent

Palliative treatment includes; stenting, radiotherapy, chemotherapy, laser therapy

(Px) 5-year survival ~5 per cent

VARICES

(P) Portal hypertension results in dilatation of veins at sites of porto-systemic anastomosis i.e. lower oesophagus, rectum, umbilicus (caput medusae)

Dilated veins project into lumen of oesophagus and are liable to haemorrhage

(Sy) Upper gastrointestinal (GI) haemorrhage, therefore haematemesis, melaena

(Si) Evidence of chronic liver disease (is there a history of alcohol abuse or cirrhosis?)

(Ix) OGD

(Rx) *Acute*:
  – resuscitate and correct possible clotting abnormalities
  – i.v. octreotide reduces bleeding
  – OGD + sclerotherapy/banding of varices
  – if unsuccessful, pass a Sengstaken–Blakemore tube (contains an inflatable balloon used to compress varices)
  – continued bleeding requires surgical decompression

Prophylaxis:
  – β-blockers to reduce portal pressure
  – OGD + sclerotherapy/banding of varices

(Px) Each bleeding episode has a mortality of ~30 per cent

ACHALASIA

P Neuromuscular disorder characterized by failure of relaxation of the lower oesophageal sphincter (LOS), together with absence of oesophageal peristalsis. May be mimicked by Chagas' disease (*Trypanosoma cruzi* infection in South America)

A Typically aged 25–60 years

Sy Dysphagia > regurgitation, chest pain, weight loss

Ix *Barium swallow*: tapering of lower oesophagus described as a 'bird's beak', together with proximal dilatation
Oesophageal manometry: reveals incomplete relaxation of LOS
OGD: exclude malignancy

Rx *Endoscopy*: pneumatic dilatation at OGD
Surgery: Heller's operation whereby the muscle of the LOS and proximal stomach is divided down to the mucosa (open or laparoscopic)

Cx Associated with malignant change in the distal oesophagus

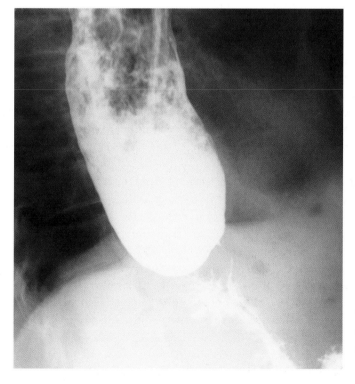

Figure 2.4 Achalasia of the oesophagus: grossly dilated oesophagus with a smooth narrowing at its lower end

PHARYNGEAL POUCH/ZENKER'S DIVERTICULUM

P Protrusion of mucosa and submucosa between two parts of the inferior pharyngeal constrictor muscle (this area of weakness is called Killian's dehiscence)

Sy Dysphagia, regurgitation, bulging or gurgling of the neck, halitosis

Si Neck swelling, halitosis, signs of aspiration pneumonia may be present

Ix Barium swallow

Rx Surgical excision of pouch, plus repair of defect in inferior constrictor

PLUMMER–VINSON/PATERSON–BROWN KELLY SYNDROME

- **P** Web: thin eccentric extension of normal oesophageal tissue
- **A** Upper oesophageal web in association with iron deficiency anaemia and dysphagia
- **Sy** Dysphagia, but web may be an incidental finding at OGD
- **Si** Those of iron deficiency anaemia i.e. koilonychia and glossitis
- **Cx** Associated with malignant change
- **Rx** Iron replacement; dilatation of web if required

STOMACH

PEPTIC ULCERS

This is covered in detail in Chapter 1 (p. 35)

Indications for surgery:

- *haemorrhage not controlled with medical therapy*:
  - duodenal ulcers – suture ligation of ulcer ± vagotomy and pyloroplasty
  - gastric ulcers – oversewing of ulcer (sometimes require resection)
- *ulcer perforation*:
  - closure with an omental patch followed by peritoneal lavage
- *ulcer producing gastric outlet obstruction*
- *malignant change*:
  - distal gastrectomy – either Billroth 1 (gastroduodenostomy) or Billroth 2 (gastrojejunostomy)

UPPER GI BLEED

This is a **surgical emergency**

- **P** Bleeding proximal to the ligament of Treitz (marks duodenojejunal flexure)
- **A** Peptic ulcer, gastritis, oesophageal varices, Mallory–Weiss tear (mucosal tear in oesophagus due to vomiting) and malignancy
- **Sy** Haematemesis (bright red or coffee-ground appearance), melaena (black motions), fresh blood per rectum (PR) (very rapid bleed)
- **Si** Assess state of shock (i.e. urine output, pulse, blood pressure [BP], conscious level). Be alert to signs of chronic liver disease. PR for melaena. Epigastric tenderness
- **Ix** *Initially*: bloods (full blood count (FBC), urea and electrolytes (U&E), coagulation, cross-match 4–6 units), urine output, electrocardiogram (ECG)
  Once stabilized: OGD to identify, treat and assess prognosis of bleeding
- **Rx** Resuscitate. Correct clotting abnormalities
  OGD allows adrenaline or sclerosant injection/diathermy/laser phototherapy/variceal banding
  Indications for surgery are Hospital Trust dependent, they include: bleeding vessel not controlled at endoscopy, continued bleeding, rebleeding and patients >60 years
- **Px** Rockall Risk Score is used to predict mortality
  Overall mortality rate: 6–10 per cent

PYLORIC STENOSIS

- **P** Hypertrophy of smooth muscle in the antrum and pylorus of the stomach
- **A** Typically presents ~4 weeks of age

Sy Non-bilious vomiting after feeding, which becomes projectile

Si Pylorus palpable as an 'olive' in epigastrium/right upper quadrant (RUQ)

Ix Ultrasound scan (USS), U&E (loss of H_2O and H^+Cl^- during vomiting)

Rx Correct dehydration and electrolyte disturbances prior to definitive treatment with Ramstedt's pyloromyotomy (incision of pylorus muscle)

GASTRIC CARCINOMA

A Incidence declining in the UK, although it remains 2nd most common cause of cancer-related death in the world (highest incidence: Japan)

Box 2.1 RISK FACTORS FOR GASTRIC CARCINOMA

- Diet (pickled/smoked foods)
- Achlorhydria e.g. atrophic gastritis, pernicious anaemia
- Blood group A
- Low social class
- *H. pylori*
- Previous gastric surgery

Sy Anorexia, weight loss, nausea, dyspepsia, dysphagia and epigastric pain, among others, are late symptoms

Si Cachexia, epigastric mass. Metastases may present with hepatomegaly or classically, a palpable Virchow's node (located in the left supraclavicular fossa)

Ix FBC may reveal anaemia

Barium meal

OGD + biopsies

CT/MRI to assess metastatic disease

Rx Total or partial gastrectomy plus lymph node resection is potentially curative. Palliative procedures centre on relieving gastric obstruction

Px 5-year survival ~20 per cent (improved in countries employing screening programmes)

SMALL INTESTINE

MECKEL'S DIVERTICULUM

P Persistence of a segment of the vitello-intestinal duct

A Rule of 2s:
  - 2 per cent population affected
  - ~2 inches long
  - ~2 feet proximal to ileocaecal valve

None of the above is **2** accurate!

Frequently contains ectopic tissue – gastric (50 per cent), pancreatic, colonic etc.

S Asymptomatic finding at laparotomy (most common)

Ulceration (due to presence of gastric mucosa), haemorrhage, small bowel obstruction, perforation, and diverticulitis

Ix Barium follow-through, technetium nuclear medicine scan, laparoscopy

(Rx) Resection of diverticulum (resection of asymptomatic Meckel's is controversial: indicated if narrow neck)

(Px) Lifetime risk of requiring surgery ~6 per cent

LARGE INTESTINE

APPENDICITIS

(P) Inflammation of the vermiform appendix (arises from caecum)

(A) Lifetime incidence ~7 per cent (rare in very young/old)
Due to bacterial infection secondary to luminal obstruction (most often a faecalith or lymphoid hyperplasia)

(Sy) Anorexia. Classically, colicky central abdominal pain (inflammation of appendix) followed by localization of pain to right iliac fossa (inflammation of overlying peritoneum)
Nausea, vomiting and constipation/diarrhoea are more variable

(Si) Low grade pyrexia, patient tries to minimize movements. Right iliac fossa (RIF) tenderness, guarding and rebound/percussion tenderness. Right-sided tenderness on PR
Rovsing's sign: RIF pain on palpation of left iliac fossa (LIF)
Differential diagnosis: ectopic pregnancy, ovarian torsion, diverticulitis, pelvic inflammatory disease, Crohn's disease, mesenteric adenitis

(Ix) Commonly ↑ white cell count (WCC) (neutrophilia) and ↑ C-reactive protein (CRP). USS and CT if uncertain of diagnosis. β-human chorionic gonadotrophin (β-HCG) to exclude ectopic pregnancy in females

(Cx) Perforation leading to either generalized peritonitis, or a localized appendix abscess. Omentum may cover inflammation resulting in an appendix mass

(Rx) Appendicectomy plus cefuroxime and metronidazole if evidence of perforation

(Px) Mortality rate <1 per cent

DIVERTICULAR DISEASE OF THE COLON

(P) Acquired outpouchings of bowel mucosa secondary to high intraluminal pressures
Most commonly affects sigmoid colon

(A) Postulated to be secondary to low-fibre Western diets

Box 2.2 IMPORTANT DEFINITIONS

- *Diverticulosis*: existence of diverticula with no inflammation
- *Diverticulitis*: inflammation of a diverticulum
- *Diverticular disease*: diverticula associated with abdominal pain and disturbed bowel habit

---

(Sy) Depend on site, severity and presence of complications
Abdominal pain (usually in LIF), fever, altered bowel habit, nausea and PR bleeding

(Si) Pyrexia. Localized tenderness, guarding and rebound/percussion tenderness (often LIF). PR for tenderness/blood

(Ix) Gastrografin enema, CT scan, sigmoidoscopy and colonoscopy.

Diverticular disease: high-fibre diet (ensure carcinoma has been excluded)
Diverticulitis:
  – mild disease treated as an outpatient with liquid diet and broad-spectrum antibiotics
  – if unable to tolerate fluids or inadequate analgesia, then admit; NBM, i.v. fluids and i.v. broad-spectrum antibiotics
  – failure to respond to medical therapy/perforation/obstruction will generally require a Hartmann's procedure, with colostomy reversal 3–6 months later

Cx Perforation, obstruction, haemorrhage, fistulae, abscess formation

STOMAS

- Surgically created opening of a tube (bowel or urinary tract) to a body surface (usually the abdomen)
- Collecting bag attaches over stoma
- Profound psychological implications for patient – involve stoma nurse early
- Stoma position decided pre-operatively (avoid umbilicus, scars and bony prominences)
- Defunctioning stomas aim to prevent digested products reaching a distal section of bowel – allow healing of an anastomosis, or resolution of infection prior to reversal
- *End ileostomy/colostomy*: single lumen of bowel
- *Loop ileostomy/colostomy*: section of bowel incised ~250° of its circumference to create two lumens
- *Double-barrel colostomy*: proximal and distal sections of bowel brought out as separate single lumens

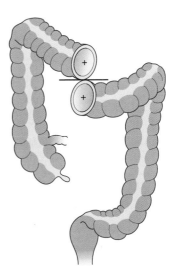

(a)   **Loop colostomy**

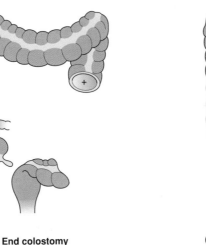

(b)   **End colostomy**

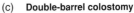

Colostomy

Mucous
fistula

(c)   **Double-barrel colostomy**

Figure 2.5 Colostomies: (a) loop colostomy; (b) end colostomy; (c) double-barrel colostomy

Ileostomy

- Stoma involving ileum
- Usually located in right lower quadrant
- Spout to prevent their irritant liquid effluent from contacting skin
  - *end ileostomy* – e.g. after total colectomy
  - *defunctioning loop ileostomy* – e.g. if concerned regarding a colonic anastomosis

Colostomy

- Stoma involving colon
- Usually located in left lower quadrant
- Flush with skin
  - *end colostomy* – e.g. after abdominoperineal resection (removal of anus and rectum for low rectal cancer)
  - *Hartmann's procedure* – distal segment of colon is left *in situ* and closed with sutures. The proximal segment is exteriorized as an end colostomy. This offers the possibility of reversal at a later date

Cx Diarrhoea and constipation

Ileostomies can result in electrolyte imbalances due to large fluid losses

Necrosis, prolapse and stenosis of stoma

Parastomal hernia

MALIGNANCY

A 2nd commonest cause of cancer-related deaths in the UK

Incidence ↑ with age

Risk factors:
- environmental: ? diet high in fat, ? alcohol, red meat
- inflammatory bowel disease
- familial adenomatous polyposis coli syndrome (FAP) and hereditary non-polyposis colon cancer (HNPCC) (see p. 118)

P Majority located in rectum and sigmoid colon (left side of colon)

Adenoma → carcinoma theory

Sy Weight loss, anorexia, change in bowel habit, blood PR, tenesmus, or abdominal pain. Symptoms of anaemia, perforation or obstruction. In general:
- *right-sided lesions*: weight loss, anaemia
- *left-sided lesions*: change of bowel habit, tenesmus, obstruction, blood PR

Si Anaemia, cachexia, palpable mass in abdomen/PR, disseminated malignancy (e.g. hepatomegaly, jaundice, lymphadenopathy). Signs of obstruction

Ix FBC: ↓ haemoglobin (Hb), ↓ mean corpuscular volume (MCV), liver function tests (LFTs) and coagulation (derangement suggests hepatic metastases), tumour markers (CEA, CA19–9), faecal occult blood

Sigmoidoscopy, colonoscopy, CT scan, barium enema

Rx Aim is surgical resection of tumour ± chemotherapy

Palliative procedures centre on relieving obstruction (e.g. stents or bypass operations)

Adjuvant radiotherapy may be employed with rectal carcinomas

(a)   (b)

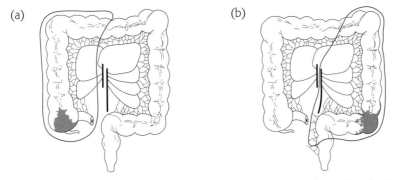

Figure 2.6 (a) Right hemicolectomy; (b) left hemicolectomy (reproduced with permission from Mortensen NJMcC in Russell RCG, Williams NS and Bulstrode CJK (eds), *Bailey & Love's Short Practice of Surgery*, 24th ed, Great Britain: Hodder Education, 2004)

Px   Depends on the stage of disease (see Table 2.1)

Table 2.1 Modified Dukes' classification of colorectal carcinoma

Stage	Pathology	5-year survival (%)
A	Confined to bowel wall (mucosa)	90
B	Growth through bowel wall (muscle)	60
C	Regional lymph node involvement	30
D	Distant metastases	5

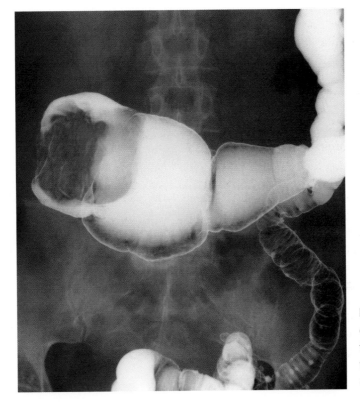

Figure 2.7 Barium enema: large polypoidal filling defect in the transverse colon due to a colonic carcinoma

FAMILIAL ADENOMATOUS POLYPOSIS COLI SYNDROME (FAP)

(A) Autosomal dominant disorder of tumour suppressor *APC* gene
Colorectal cancer develops in all patients if no treatment
(P) Characterized by hundreds/thousands adenomatous polyps throughout the colon
(Rx) Prophylactic total colectomy, excision of rectum and formation of ileoanal pouch

HEREDITARY NON-POLYPOSIS COLON CANCER (HNPCC)

- Autosomal dominant disorder of DNA mismatch repair system
- Develop mainly right-sided carcinomas
- Very few colorectal polyps develop (hence the name)

SURGICAL ASPECTS OF INFLAMMATORY BOWEL DISEASE

Ulcerative colitis

- Surgically curable disease (it is limited to the colon)
- *Operations*: proctocolectomy and ileostomy versus total colectomy and ileoanal pouch
- *Indications*: failure to control disease with medication, unacceptable drug side-effects, evidence of dysplasia or strictures, toxic megacolon

Crohn's disease

- Surgery is not curative – aim to avoid surgical intervention
- *Operations*: segmental resection, temporary colostomy/ileostomy
- *Indications*:
  - failure to control disease with medication, strictures and perforation, perianal fistulae and abscesses.
  - temporary colostomy/ileostomy may allow healing of perianal fistulae/abscesses

ANAL AND PERIANAL DISEASE

HAEMORRHOIDS

(A) Affect 50 per cent of population aged over 50 years
Predisposing conditions: straining with defaecation, pregnancy
(P) Displacement and dilatation of one or more anal cushions (vascular tissue)
Classified into grades I–IV:

Box 2.3 CLASSIFICATION OF HAEMORRHOIDS

- *Grade I*: bleed only
- *Grade II*: prolapse but spontaneously reduce
- *Grade III*: prolapse and require manual replacement
- *Grade IV*: permanently prolapsed

(Sy) Painless bright red PR bleeding, perianal lump, pruritus ani
(Si) Visible prolapsed haemorrhoids and anaemia (if bleeding is brisk)
Examine abdomen for masses

Ix PR (haemorrhoids are not palpable), proctoscopy (visualize haemorrhoids), sigmoidoscopy (to exclude higher pathology)

Rx Increase dietary fibre and fluid intake + stop straining at stool
Grade I–III: sclerosant injection/banding/cryotherapy in outpatients
Grade IV: haemorrhoidectomy (also indicated if above measures fail)

Cx Strangulation; blood supply to a prolapsed haemorrhoid is restricted due to contraction of the anal sphincter, resulting in pain and swelling. May become thrombosed (extremely painful)

PERIANAL HAEMATOMA

P Rupture of a perianal subcutaneous blood vessel

Sy Acute onset of perianal pain after straining at stool

Si Blue/black bulge at the anal margin

Rx Resolves spontaneously. Incision indicated only for pain relief

FISSURE IN ANO

P Painful tear in the anal epithelium ± mucosa
Associated with hypertonicity of internal sphincter
Majority occur in posterior midline

A Thought to be secondary to passage of a hard stool

Sy Severe pain during and after bowel motions, bright red PR bleeding

Si Fissure, sentinel pile

Ix PR may be impossible due to pain

Rx *Conservative*: dietary fibre and stool softeners
Medical: glyceryl trinitrate (GTN) cream (relaxes internal sphincter), botox
Surgery: indicated for failed medical treatment or chronic fissure – anal stretch (now rarely performed), lateral sphincterotomy

Cx If fissure occurs off midline or suspicious history, exclude other diagnoses e.g. Crohn's disease, AIDS, carcinoma

ANORECTAL ABSCESS

P Infection originating in cryptoglandular epithelium lining the anal canal spreads to surrounding soft tissues, with subsequent abscess formation
Location: perianal 60 per cent, ischiorectal 20 per cent, intersphincteric 5 per cent, supralevator 4 per cent (see Fig. 2.8)

A Predisposing factors to exclude: Crohn's, diabetes, immunosuppression, TB, cancer

Sy Anal or rectal pain, often worse on defecation. Fevers/rigors

Si Visible erythematous, fluctuant mass

Ix Fluctuant tender mass on PR. Examination under anaesthesia (EUA). May require CT/MRI of intersphincteric and supralevator abscesses

Rx Early surgical drainage with healing by secondary intention

Cx Fistula formation in 7–40 per cent of patients

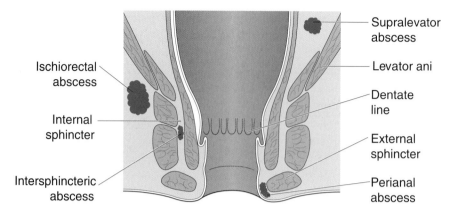

Figure 2.8 Locations of peri-anal abscesses

FISTULA IN ANO

P   An abnormal connection between a primary opening inside the anal canal and a secondary opening in the perianal skin

A   Majority form secondary to a perianal abscess (again remember to rule out Crohn's, carcinoma, TB etc.)

Parks' classification: intersphincteric 70 per cent, trans-sphincteric 25 per cent, suprasphincteric 5 per cent and extrasphincteric <1 per cent

Goodsall's rule: imagine a transverse line through the anus in the lithotomy position. Fistulae with an external opening anterior to this line will follow a straight line to the anus. Fistulae with an opening posterior to this line follow a curved course to open in the midline

Sy   History of anorectal abscess. Perianal discharge and pain persist

Si   External opening on perineum ± visible discharge

Ix   PR (may palpate primary opening). MRI to evaluate complex fistulae. EUA

Rx   Laying open of fistula in intersphincteric and low trans-sphincteric fistulae (do not involve internal/external sphincter)

High fistulae require two-stage surgery involving placement of a seton (a suture) through the fistula to promote scar tissue and maintain sphincter integrity

Cx   Recurrence. Faecal incontinence post-operatively

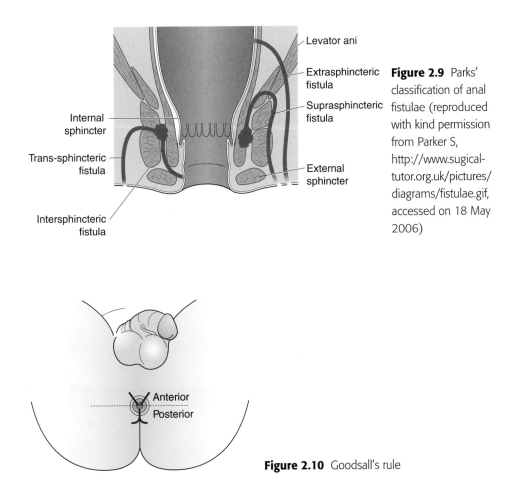

Figure 2.9 Parks' classification of anal fistulae (reproduced with kind permission from Parker S, http://www.sugical-tutor.org.uk/pictures/diagrams/fistulae.gif, accessed on 18 May 2006)

Figure 2.10 Goodsall's rule

PILONIDAL SINUS

 Hair-containing sinus in the sacro-coccygeal area (majority in natal cleft)

A Controversial: hair follicle inflammation with subsequent trapping of hairs, which act as foreign bodies, thus producing chronic inflammation

Risk factors: male, hirsute, obese, occupations involving prolonged sitting (classically taxi/lorry drivers)

Sy Asymptomatic, or pain, purulent discharge

Si Visible tracts ± purulent discharge, tenderness, fluctuance

Rx *Conservative*:
- local hygiene and shaving

Surgery:
- incision and drainage of abscess/sinus
- recurrence may require wide skin excision + skin flaps

RECTAL PROLAPSE

P Two distinct clinical entities:
- *full-thickness* – prolapse of all layers of rectal wall through anus
- *mucosal* – prolapse of rectal mucosa through anus

A Majority of patients are women (often multiparous). Also children <3 years, Down's syndrome, mentally handicapped

Sy Palpable mass, faecal incontinence, PR bleeding

Si Protruding rectal mass (ask patient to bear down), reduced sphincter tone on PR, evidence of ulceration

Ix Sweat test to exclude cystic fibrosis in children
Sigmoidoscopy to examine rectal mucosa for ulceration or other contributing disease

Rx Acutely, reduce with gentle digital pressure
Definitive surgical repair is either via a perineal (e.g. Delorme's procedure) or abdominal (open or laparoscopic rectopexy) approach

ANAL CARCINOMA

A Uncommon tumour (incidence ~300 per year)
Predisposing factors include anal warts, increased incidence in homosexuals, pre-existing anal warts (human papillomavirus [HPV])

P 80 per cent are squamous cell carcinomas

Sy Change in bowel habit, pain, bleeding, palpable mass

Rx Radiotherapy is now the mainstay of treatment

HIRSCHSPRUNG'S DISEASE

P Absence of parasympathetic ganglion cells in the rectum or colon

A Commonly males

S Presents as acute obstruction with failure to pass meconium in the neonate, or chronic constipation in older children

BOWEL OBSTRUCTION

P *Simple obstruction*: occlusion of bowel without vascular compromise
Strangulation: occlusion of bowel with vascular compromise

Si Absent bowel sounds, constant localized pain and peritonism, ↑WCC

Box 2.4 GENERAL CLASSIFICATION OF CAUSES OF BOWEL OBSTRUCTION

- *Intraluminal*:
  - foreign body
  - impacted faeces/food
  - intussusception
  - gallstones
- *Bowel wall lesions*:
  - tumours
  - strictures
  - Crohn's disease
  - diverticulitis
- *Extrinsic*:
  - adhesions
  - hernias
  - volvulus
  - external compression

LARGE INTESTINE

 Commonly carcinoma, sigmoid/caecal volvulus (twisting of bowel around its mesenteric attachment)

Box 2.5 THE FOUR CLASSIC SIGNS OF COMPLETE BOWEL OBSTRUCTION

1   Absolute constipation (no passage of flatus or faeces)
2   Colicky abdominal pain
3   Abdominal distension
4   Vomiting (often late or absent)

 As in Box 2.5; note that passage of flatus suggests partial obstruction
Discomfort, dehydration and tachycardia
Abdomen:
– distended, generalized tenderness, evidence of scars or masses
– tinkling bowel sounds.
PR: empty rectum, faecal impaction, mass, blood

Ix *Bloods*: minor ↑ WCC, dehydration on U&Es (third space losses)
Erect CXR: air under the diaphragm indicates perforation
AXR (abdominal X-ray): distended large bowel (>5 cm diameter), identified by its peripheral position and haustral folds (partially cross lumen)
Gastrografin enema: to identify level/cause of obstruction
CT scan: to identify level/cause of obstruction

Rx NBM, nasogastric tube (NGT) insertion and i.v. fluid resuscitation – 'drip and suck'
Endoscopic reduction of sigmoid volvulus (allows planned definitive surgical procedure)
Removal of obstruction and resection of accompanying non-viable bowel, followed by delayed anastomosis due to invariable faecal contamination (i.e. temporary colostomy)

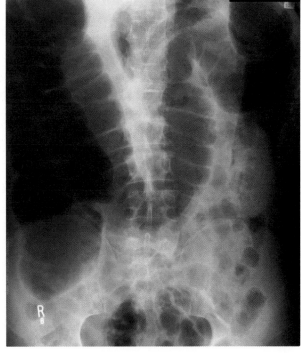

Figure 2.11 Large bowel obstruction: gas is seen in the large bowel up to the mid-descending colon

SMALL INTESTINE

(A) *Common causes*:
- – adhesions (fibrous bands between loops of bowel secondary to previous abdominal surgery)
- – hernias

(Sy) Absolute constipation may be a late feature
Vomiting (occurs early), periumbilical colicky pain, distension (less than large bowel)

(Si) Discomfort, dehydration and tachycardia
Abdomen : distended, generalized tenderness, evidence of scars, hernias or masses
Tinkling bowel sounds
PR: empty rectum, blood

(Ix) *Bloods*: minor $\uparrow$ WCC, dehydration on U&Es
Erect CXR: air under the diaphragm indicates perforation
AXR : distended small bowel (>2.5 cm diameter), identified by its central position and valvulae conniventes (completely cross lumen)
CT scan: identify level/cause of obstruction
Barium follow-through: to identify level/cause of obstruction

(Rx) Trial of NBM, NGT insertion and i.v. fluid resuscitation
Evidence of strangulation, or failure of conservative measures requires laparotomy to remove the cause of obstruction and resect non-viable bowel (usually with primary anastomosis)

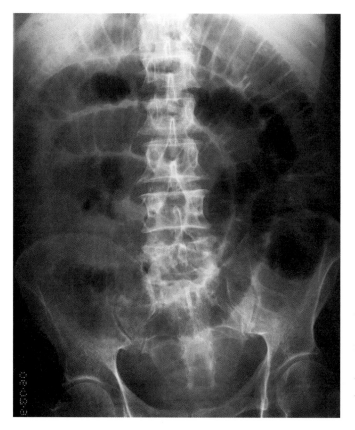

Figure 2.12 Small bowel obstruction: multiple dilated small bowel loops with absence of gas in the large bowel; note the small bowel folds (valvulae conniventes) traverse the entire thickness of the small bowel

INTUSSUSCEPTION

(P) Telescoping of one portion of bowel into an immediately adjacent segment. Subsequent restriction of blood supply and oedema of bowel wall rapidly leads to obstruction and potentially gangrene/perforation

(A) Most common in those aged 3–12 months

(Sy) Paroxysmal colicky abdominal pain, vomiting and redcurrant jelly stools

(Si) Pale, palpable sausage-shaped mass, redcurrant jelly on PR

(Rx) Reduction with air enema. If this fails, reduction at laparotomy is required

(a)
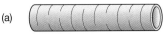
Normal

(b)
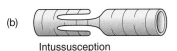
Intussusception

Figure 2.13 Intussusception: (a) normal intestine; (b) intussusception

PSEUDO-OBSTRUCTION/ILEUS

(P) Functional bowel obstruction due to reduced motility

(A) Metabolic disturbances, anticholinergics, intra-operative bowel manipulation

(Sy) As per large/small bowel obstruction

(Si) As per large/small bowel obstruction *except* bowel sounds are absent

(Ix) U&Es. AXR and Gastrografin swallow/enema reveal dilated bowel with no evidence of mechanical obstruction

(Rx) Withhold drugs which inhibit GI mobility. Correct electrolyte abnormalities with i.v. fluids. NGT. Analgesia

Pro-kinetics such as oral metoclopramide and erythromycin, or i.v. neostigmine may be effective

Decompression may be attempted via colonoscopy

HERNIAS

(P) Protrusion of a viscus or part of a viscus through its containing cavity into an abnormal position

---

Box 2.6 COMMON TERMS USED TO DESCRIBE HERNIAS

- *Reducible*: can push back into original cavity
- *Irreducible/incarcerated*: unable to push back into original cavity
- *Obstructed*: bowel contents unable to pass through hernia
- *Strangulated*: blood supply of contents is occluded

(A) Abdominal wall hernias occur at sites of inherent weakness. Operations, advancing age, obesity and malnutrition result in further loss of muscular strength

Raised intra-abdominal pressure is also a risk factor e.g. chronic cough or constipation, urinary obstruction, heavy lifting

(Sy) Lump, pain or symptoms of complication i.e. obstruction or strangulation

(Si) Lump at recognized site with an expansile cough impulse

Scars

A tense, tender and erythematous lump together with signs of intestinal obstruction suggests strangulation

(Ix) USS if unsure of diagnosis

(Rx) Surgical repair unless risk of strangulation is low (e.g. large defect in containing cavity). In general, surgery involves excision of the hernial sac (herniotomy) and repair of the hernial defect (herniorrhaphy)

(Cx) Obstruction and strangulation

INGUINAL HERNIA

(P) Protrusion of a viscus through the inguinal canal

(A) ♂ > ♀

The inguinal canal is an oblique passage through the inferior part of the anterior abdominal wall. Contents – spermatic cord (♂), round ligament (♀) and ilioinguinal nerve (♂♀)

Table 2.2 Borders of the inguinal canal

	Lateral	Medial
Floor	Inguinal ligament	Inguinal ligament and lacunar ligament
Roof	Internal oblique and transversus abdominis	Internal oblique and transversus abdominis
Anterior wall	External oblique aponeurosis and internal oblique	External oblique aponeurosis
Posterior wall	Transversalis fascia	Transversalis fascia

Internal ring:
– U-shaped condensation of transversalis fascia which allows passage of cord from abdomen into inguinal canal
– lies at midpoint of inguinal ligament (halfway between pubic tubercle and anterior superior iliac spine [ASIS]), lateral to inferior epigastric vessels
External ring:
– formed by two crura of external oblique which allows spermatic cord to leave the inguinal canal and enter the scrotum
– lies just above and medial to the pubic tubercle
Indirect inguinal hernias enter canal via the internal ring (65 per cent)
Direct inguinal hernias enter canal via a defect in the posterior wall medial to the internal ring (35 per cent)

(Si) Hernia originates above and medial to the pubic tubercle
Once reduced, digital pressure over the internal ring will prevent an indirect hernia from reappearing when the patient is asked to cough. Reappearance of the hernia during this manoeuvre suggests a direct hernia (NB this is not an accurate test – accurate determination can only be made operatively)

Rx *Conservative*: truss (like a corset) is prescribed in patients whose comorbidity excludes them from operative repair
Surgery: laparoscopic or open. Defect repaired with sutures or mesh

FEMORAL HERNIA

P Protrusion of a viscus through the femoral canal
Canal connects superiorly with abdomen via femoral ring

A ♀ > ♂ (NB overall inguinal hernias > femoral hernias in women)

Si Hernia originates below and lateral to the pubic tubercle

Rx Always require surgical repair as hernia is prone to obstruction and strangulation against the sharp lacunar ligament (medial border of canal)

INCISIONAL HERNIA

P Protrusion of a viscus through the scar of a previous operation/injury
Skin remains intact

A *Pre-operative*: elderly, respiratory disease, anaemia, obesity, uraemia, jaundice, diabetes, malnutrition, malignancy, steroids or cytotoxics
Intra-operative: type of incision/sutures, surgical technique
Post-operative: wound infection, ischaemia, abdominal distension, chronic cough

Sy Cosmetic appearance (usually have a large neck, therefore low risk of strangulation)

Si Hernia with overlying scar

Rx Truss if unsuitable (or unwilling) to have surgery
Surgical closure of defect with sutures ± mesh

Cx Recurrence of hernia after repair

GALLSTONES AND RELATED DISORDERS

A Affects 12 per cent men and 24 per cent women

P Bile contains cholesterol, bile salts and lecithin
Three main types of stone: cholesterol, pigment, and mixed

Rx May be asymptomatic

Cx Complications best considered in relation to position (see Fig. 2.14)

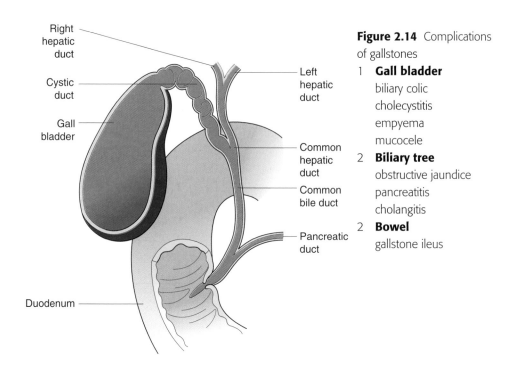

Right hepatic duct
Cystic duct
Gall bladder
Left hepatic duct
Common hepatic duct
Common bile duct
Pancreatic duct
Duodenum

Figure 2.14 Complications of gallstones
1 **Gall bladder**
   biliary colic
   cholecystitis
   empyema
   mucocele
2 **Biliary tree**
   obstructive jaundice
   pancreatitis
   cholangitis
2 **Bowel**
   gallstone ileus

BILIARY COLIC

- **P** Due to impaction of stone in gall bladder neck or cystic duct
- **Sy** RUQ colicky pain (± radiation to tip of right scapula), vomiting
- **Si** Tender RUQ
- **Ix** Bloods (FBC, LFTs, U&Es, amylase), USS
- **Rx** *Conservative*: NBM, i.v. fluids, opiate analgesia
  Surgery: laparoscopic (rarely open) cholecystectomy at 6–12 weeks when biliary tree less inflamed

CHOLECYSTITIS

- **P** An impacted stone obstructing the gall bladder outlet may result in infection of the accumulating bile
- **Sy** Constant RUQ pain (± referred pain radiating to tip of right scapula)
  Fever and vomiting
- **Si** Pyrexia, tenderness, rebound and guarding in RUQ
  Murphy's sign: patient catches breath on inspiration when two fingers are placed in RUQ (valid if negative in left upper quadrant [LUQ])
- **Ix** FBC (↑WCC), USS (gallstones, thickened gall bladder wall, pericholecystic fluid)
- **Rx** *Conservative*: NBM, analgesia, i.v. fluids and antibiotics (e.g. cefuroxime and metronidazole)
  Surgery: laparoscopic (rarely open) cholecystectomy (72 h or 6–12 weeks)
- **Cx** Chronic cholecystitis, mucocele (distends with bile), empyema (distends with pus), gangrene and perforation

GALLSTONE OBSTRUCTIVE JAUNDICE

P   Gallstone impacts in, and obstructs common bile duct

Sy   Jaundice, pale stools, dark urine, pruritus

Symptoms of biliary colic or painless

Si   Jaundice ± tenderness RUQ

Ix   Bloods (↑ alkaline phosphatase [ALP], gamma glutamyl transferase [GGT], unconjugated bilirubin)

USS, endoscopic retrograde cholangiopancreatography (ERCP), magnetic resonance cholangiopancreatography (MRCP) to image biliary tree

Rx   *Endoscopy*: ERCP allows stone removal/sphincterotomy/stent placement

Surgery: open bile duct exploration, cholecystectomy 6–12 weeks

Cx   Ascending cholangitis

ASCENDING CHOLANGITIS

P   Gallstone impacted in the common bile duct (CBD) results in infection of the biliary system

Sy   Pale stools, dark urine and pruritus

Charcot's triad:

1. jaundice
2. fever
3. RUQ pain

Si   Pyrexia, RUQ tenderness and rigors

Ix   Bloods (↑ WCC in addition to a picture of obstructive jaundice), USS, ERCP, MRCP

Rx   *Conservative*: NBM, analgesia, i.v. fluids and antibiotics (e.g. cefuroxime and metronidazole)

Endoscopy: ERCP allows stone removal/sphincterotomy/stent placement

Surgery: open bile duct exploration, cholecystectomy 6–12 weeks

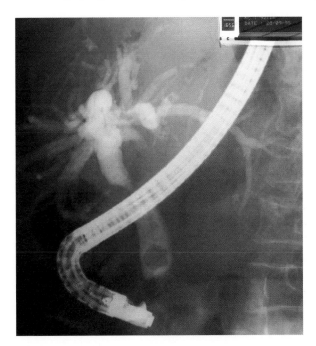

Figure 2.15 ERCP showing a lobulated filling defect in the common bile duct from a calculus

GALLSTONE ILEUS

(P) Gallstone erodes through into the duodenum

May cause a mechanical bowel obstruction

GALL BLADDER CARCINOMA

(A) Rare, 80 per cent have gallstones

(Sy) Abdominal pain, nausea and vomiting, weight loss

(Rx) If possible, operative resection

(Px) Very poor

CHOLANGIOCARCINOMA

(P) Malignancy of the biliary tree

Intra- or extra-hepatic

(A) Associated with primary sclerosing cholangitis (and hence inflammatory bowel disease [IBD])

(Sy) As with obstructive jaundice + dull abdominal pain, weight loss

(Si) Palpable gall bladder, abdominal mass, hepatomegaly

(Ix) USS, MRI, CT

(Rx) *Palliation*: stents, radiotherapy and chemotherapy

Surgery: 10 per cent may be suitable for curative resection

PANCREAS

ACUTE PANCREATITIS

(P) Inflammation of exocrine pancreas

(A) Most common (>95 per cent): gallstones/alcohol

Other causes: tumours, viruses (mumps), thiazide diuretics, hyperlipidaemia, hypercalcaemia, ERCP (iatrogenic)

(Sy) Severe epigastric pain (radiates to back), nausea, vomiting

(Si) ↑ heart rate (HR), ↑ temperature, ↓ BP, abdominal tenderness, ↓ bowel sounds (secondary to ileus)

Generalized tenderness and guarding

Grey–Turner's sign: flank discolouration

Cullen's sign: periumbilical discolouration

(Ix) Serum amylase >1000 IU/ml, FBC, U&E, LFT, arterial blood gases (ABG), USS, CT

(Rx) Analgesia, i.v. fluids, O_2, naso-jejunal feeding (to avoid pancreatic stimulation), ERCP if gallstone obstructing bile duct

(Cx) Pseudocyst (fluid collection in lesser sac), abscess, respiratory distress, renal failure, chronic pancreatitis

(Px) Depends on severity of attack (see Box 2.7, Ranson criteria)

Box 2.7 RANSON CRITERIA IN ACUTE PANCREATITIS

- *At admission or diagnosis*:
  - age $>$ 55 years
  - WCC $>$ 16 000/mm^3
  - glucose $>$ 11 mmol/L
  - lactate dehydrogenase $>$ 350 IU/L
  - aspartate transaminase (AST) $>$ 600 IU/L
- *During initial 48 h*:
  - haematocrit fall $>$ 10 per cent
  - calcium $<$ 2 mmol/L
  - Pao$_2$ (arterial partial pressure of oxygen) $<$ 8 kPa
  - BE (base excess) $>$ -4 mmol/L
  - urea increase $>$ 1.8 mmol/L
  - fluid sequestration $>$ 6 L
- *Prognosis*:
  - 0–2 criteria $<$ 5 per cent mortality
  - 3–4 criteria 20 per cent mortality
  - 5–6 criteria 40 per cent mortality
  - 7–8 criteria 100 per cent mortality

CHRONIC PANCREATITIS

P Long-term pathological process of pancreatic fibrosis + calcification

A Majority due to chronic alcohol use

Sy Chronic abdominal pain relieved by opiates, fat malabsorption → steatorrhoea

Ix Serum amylase (may be normal)

CT: pancreatic calcification

Pancreatic function tests: endocrine/exocrine insufficiency

Rx Stop alcohol consumption

Pancreatic enzyme supplementation for malabsorption

Analgesia (may require coeliac plexus block)

Surgical resection if pain refractory to opioid analgesics

PANCREATIC CARCINOMA

A Incidence ↑ in UK

Associated with chronic pancreatitis, diabetes, and smoking

Patients are typically 50–70 years of age

P Mostly ductal adenocarcinomas, occurring in head of pancreas

Sy Abdominal/back pain, weight loss, anorexia

Si Painless jaundice, thrombophlebitis migrans (tender nodules in blood vessels), palpable gall bladder, ascites

Courvoisier's Law: 'if in the presence of jaundice the gall bladder is palpable, then the jaundice is unlikely to be due to stones'

Ix Bloods (obstructive jaundice, ↑ CA19–9), USS, CT, ERCP (plus cytological brushings)

Rx *Palliative*: analgesia, biliary stents, bypass surgery (for bowel obstruction)

Curative: <10 per cent suitable for Whipple's pancreatoduodenectomy

Px Poor, 10 per cent 1-year survival

Rare hormone-secreting pancreatic tumours

- *Insulinoma*: recurrent hypoglycaemic attacks
- *Glucagonoma*: diabetes, dermatitis
- VIPoma (vasoactive intestinal peptide-oma): watery diarrhoea
- *Gastrinoma*: recurrent GI ulceration (Zollinger–Ellison syndrome)

SPLEEN

SPLENIC RUPTURE

P Highly vascular organ
A Most commonly injured organ in blunt abdominal trauma
Risk of rupture increased in infectious mononucleosis, malaria and haematological malignancies
Sy *Stable patients*: asymptomatic or LUQ pain
Unstable patients: abdominal distension, tenderness and shock
Ix CT (graded I–V)
Rx Conservative non-operative management is preferable
Ongoing haemorrhage requires angiographic embolization of vessels, or splenectomy (immunize against haemophilus, meningococcus and pneumococcus infection prior to discharge)

SKIN

SEBORRHOEIC KERATOSIS

A Common benign tumour in elderly
Sy Cosmetic, catch on clothing
Si Brown/yellow round to oval lesion ± greasy with well-demarcated border
Rx Shave biopsy to exclude melanoma or for cosmetic reasons

SOLAR KERATOSIS

A Most common sun-related growth
Fair/blonde/red haired are at most risk
Sy Single lesion in sun-exposed skin (typically face, ears, dorsum of hands) which progresses/becomes multiple
Si Generally a flat lesion with a rough/scaly surface
Ix Biopsy suspicious/non-responding lesions
Rx Educate about minimizing sun exposure and sunscreen
Cryotherapy. For large areas use topical 5-fluorouracil (5-FU)
Cx Potential to undergo malignant change

KERATOACANTHOMA

P Low-grade malignancy
Sy Rapidly growing nodule with central crateriform ulceration
Rx Will resolve spontaneously (residual scarring)
Excision biopsy to exclude squamous cell carcinoma (SCC) and minimize scarring

SEBACEOUS CYST (EPIDERMOID CYST)

P Mostly found in hair-bearing areas

Sy Asymptomatic, mobile, firm to fluctuant dome shaped lesion ± central punctum
Foul-smelling toothpaste-like discharge

Si Tethered to overlying skin

Rx Excision (failure to completely remove sac may result in recurrence)

DERMOID CYST

P Cystic swellings

A *Inclusion dermoids*: embryological origin
Implantation dermoids: secondary to penetrating injury (introduces epidermal cells subcutaneously)

Rx Excision

LIPOMA

A Most common benign soft tissue tumour in adults

Sy Cosmetic. Multiple and tender lipomas – Dercum's disease

Si Smooth and fluctuant

Rx Excision for cosmetic reasons – no malignant transformation risk

NECROTIZING FASCIITIS

P Infection spreads from subcutaneous tissue along fascial planes
Involvement of scrotum and penis: Fournier's gangrene

A Usually polymicrobial infection (classically involves group A β-haemolytic streptococcus)
Infected needle, abscesses, open fractures, surgery, or idiopathic

Sy Fever, erythema ± vesicle formation

Si Initially similar to cellulitis, septic, rapidly advancing erythema ± painless ulcers

Ix Bloods ($\uparrow$WCC, $\downarrow$Na$^+$), CT

Rx Intensive therapy unit (ITU)
Broad-spectrum i.v. antibiotics. Bold surgical resection down to healthy tissue – reassess daily

Px Mortality ~25 per cent

MALIGNANT SKIN LESIONS

BASAL CELL CARCINOMA (BCC)

A Most common skin cancer, caused by sun exposure, radiation

P Typically occur on head and neck
Slow growing and locally destructive (does not metastasize)

Sy Non-healing skin lesion which may bleed

Si Raised pearly nodule with rolled edge. Often crossed by fine blood vessels

Ix Biopsy

Rx Radiotherapy/curettage/excision depending on characteristics

Cx Increased risk of developing further BCC. Metastasis extremely unusual

SQUAMOUS CELL CARCINOMA

(A) Second most common skin cancer
Arises in sun-exposed skin
More common in fair/blonde/red hair types
If arising in area of chronic inflammation – Marjolin's ulcer

(Sy) New skin lesion: asymptomatic/itch/bleed/pain

(Si) Ulcerated firm pink/flesh-coloured irregular lesion. May be a background of multiple solar keratoses

(Ix) Biopsy

(Rx) Resection

(Cx) 2–6 per cent metastasize

BOWEN'S DISEASE

(P) SCC *in situ*

(A) Sun exposure, arsenic, HPV 16

(S) Asymptomatic, enlarging, scaly erythematous plaque

(Sy) Cryotherapy, topical 5-FU, or surgical excision

(Cx) 5 per cent progress to invasive SCC

MALIGNANT MELANOMA

(P) Malignancy of melanocytes
Four main subtypes: superficial spreading, nodular, lentigo maligna and acral lentiginous

(A) 4 per cent of skin cancers but causes most skin cancer-related deaths
Arise *de novo* or in pre-existing melanocytic naevi (moles)
Risk factors: fair skin, sun exposure (legs ♀, arms and trunk ♂)

(S) Changing mole. Remember **ABCD**:

Box 2.8 WORRYING FEATURES OF A MOLE

- **A**symmetry
- **B**order irregularity
- **C**olour variation
- **D**iameter >6mm

 Excisional biopsy to stage tumour → Breslow depth (or Clark level)

(Rx) Primary prevention with sun exposure avoidance and sunscreen
Surgical resection ± lymph node dissection

(Cx) Metastases

(Px) Correlates with Breslow depth (i.e. depth of invasion)
  – <0.76 mm: 99 per cent 5-year survival
  – >4mm: 25 per cent 5-year survival

VASCULAR SURGERY

ARTERIAL OCCLUSIVE DISEASE

LOWER LIMB

P Most common cause atherosclerosis
Sudden onset suggests embolic disease

A *Fixed risk factors:* age, male sex, diabetes, family history of early atherosclerosis
Modifiable risk factors: smoking, hyperlipidaemia, hypertension

Sy Intermittent claudication, rest pain, ulcers

Si Cold limb, pallor, absent/weak pulses, muscle weakness, reduced sensation

---

Box 2.9 SIX 'P'S OF CRITICAL ISCHAEMIA

- Pain
- Pallor
- Perishing with cold
- Pulselessness
- Paraesthesiae
- Paralysis

Ix ECG (atrial fibrillation), urinalysis, FBC, lipid profile, USS, arteriography, magnetic resonance angiography (MRA)
Ankle-brachial pressure index (ABPI):
  – ≥1 = normal,
  – 0.9–0.6 = claudication,
  – 0.6–0.3 = rest pain,
  – <0.3 = critical ischaemia

Rx *Conservative:* smoking cessation, control of diabetes, hypertension and hyperlipidaemia, aspirin, exercise programme
Operative: angioplasty ± stent, open endarterectomy, bypass
Embolus: anticoagulation, thrombolysis, embolectomy

Cx Gangrene, renal failure, compartment syndrome

Px Variable, poor if risk factors not modified
Embolism: good if treated within 24 h of onset; source of embolus must be sought

---

INFORMATION BOX: ABPI

- ABPI: ankle brachial pressure index is measured by taking blood pressures from the ankle and arm and calculating the ratio.
- Usually BP is higher in the leg than the arm.
- If blood flow to the leg is impaired, leg BP drops below arm BP: the greater the drop the worse the blood flow.
- Caution is needed in diabetes where calcification of vessels can give falsely high readings.

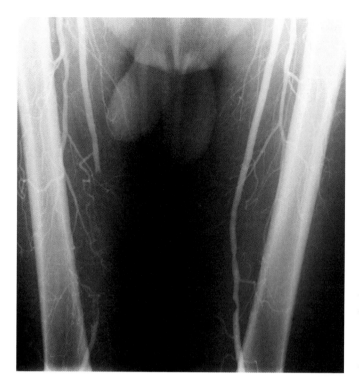

Figure 2.16 Angiogram showing a femoral artery embolus: filling defect in the right superficial femoral artery, its upper border having a convex protrusion on the contrast column

INTERMITTENT CLAUDICATION

P   Ischaemic muscle pain brought on by exercise and relieved by rest
      Most common site is the calf
S   Aorto-iliac disease causes thigh/buttock pain
      Rest pain occurs in the foot when perfusion is inadequate for basal metabolic needs
      Rest pain most common at night due to elevated feet and ↓ BP during sleep

LERICHE'S SYNDROME

P   Combination of buttock claudication and impotence – caused by aorto-iliac disease
Rx As above with conservative or operative therapy depending on patient choice, fitness, and overall prognosis

BUERGER'S DISEASE

P   Also known as thromboangiitis obliterans
      Inflammation and occlusion of medium-sized arteries
A   Common in male smokers, much younger age of onset than atherosclerosis
Rx Patients must give up smoking or risk developing irreversible damage to arterial tree
Px Worse prognosis than atherosclerosis

CAROTID DISEASE

P   Atherosclerosis common at bifurcation/internal carotid artery origin
      Stroke is third commonest cause of death in UK
      80 per cent of strokes are ischaemic
Sy Amaurosis fugax (temporary unilateral blindness), transient ischaemic attack (TIA), stroke

(Si) Carotid bruit

(Ix) FBC, U&E, glucose, lipid profile, duplex USS, MRA, carotid angiography (less common recently)

(Rx) *All patients*: smoking cessation, control of diabetes, hypertension and hyperlipidaemia, aspirin
Symptomatic patients with 70–99 per cent stenosis: carotid endarterectomy under local anaesthetic (LA) or general anaesthetic (GA)
Important complications of endarterectomy include stroke and death

(Px) Surgical benefit proven for those with symptomatic/severe stenosis

MESENTERIC DISEASE

(P) Due to either atherosclerosis or embolus

(Sy) *Ischaemia:* mesenteric angina (abdominal pain after eating), fear of eating
Infarction: abdominal pain, shock, rectal bleeding

(Si) Weight loss, abdominal tenderness, mass if bowel infarcted

(Ix) FBC, U&E, glucose, ABG, erect CXR, mesenteric angiography

(Rx) *Ischaemia:* arterial bypass sometimes possible
Infarction: bowel resection

(Px) Depends on extent of affected bowel; total mesenteric infarction usually fatal

UPPER LIMB

(P) Atherosclerosis uncommon, embolus more common
Buerger's disease may affect upper limbs

(S) As for lower limb acute ischaemia

(Ix) Often clinical diagnosis, may use duplex USS, arteriography

(Rx) Anticoagulation, thrombolysis, embolectomy

(Px) Good if treated within 24 h of onset, source of embolus must be sought

RAYNAUD'S PHENOMENON/DISEASE

(A) Common

(P) Intermittent spasm of small arteries and arterioles of hands and feet
Raynaud's *disease* is idiopathic and occurs in females
Raynaud's *phenomenon* is due to a range of causes e.g. connective tissue disorder

(Sy) Characteristic colour changes in hands, often triggered by cold exposure
Classically occur in the following stages:
1. white (ischaemic)
2. blue (cyanosed), and finally
3. red (hyperaemic)

(Si) May be none, necrotic areas on digits

(Ix) Exclude other causes of ischaemia e.g. cervical rib, subclavian stenosis, Buerger's disease

(Rx) *Supportive:* smoking cessation, keep hands and feet warm
Medical: vasodilator drugs (rarely successful)
Surgery: sympathectomy (good result but usually short-lived), amputation of necrotic digits if disease is severe

ULCERS

ARTERIAL

P   Caused by chronic ischaemia
    Large vessel disease (e.g. atherosclerosis) or small vessel (e.g. diabetes)
    Usually on toes or over pressure areas

Sy   Pain at rest (venous ulcers are classically painless)

Si   Punched-out edge, sloughy base, may be very deep, poor peripheral pulses, other
    signs of ischaemia in affected limb (pallor, cyanosis)

Ix   As for ischaemic limb, biopsy

Rx   As for ischaemic limb. May need debridement and skin grafting after
    revascularization of limb. Amputation for uncontrollable pain

Px   Poor as often a sign of end-stage vascular disease

VENOUS

A   Common in patients with venous reflux disease
    May be a history of deep vein thrombosis (DVT) (so called post-thrombotic limb)

P   Occurs with both deep and superficial reflux
    Usually preceded by chronic venous skin changes e.g. venous eczema,
    lipodermatosclerosis (chronic fibrosis of skin/fat secondary to extravasation of red
    blood cells)
    Usually in the gaiter area (see Fig. 2.17)

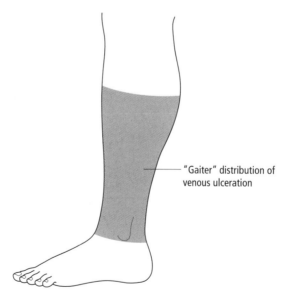

"Gaiter" distribution of venous ulceration

Figure 2.17 Gaiter distribution of venous ulceration

Sy   Pain, mainly when dressings are applied, little pain at rest

Si   Sloping edge, granulation tissue and fibrotic tissue in base, usually shallow, usually
    venous skin changes in surrounding tissue, often varicose veins in affected limb

Ix   Exclude ischaemia, venous duplex USS, biopsy

Rx   *Conservative*: 4-layer compression bandaging and/or hosiery

       Surgical: correction of superficial venous reflux, debridement and skin grafting

Px   Good, may require lifelong compression hosiery

MARJOLIN'S ULCER

P   Squamous cell carcinoma in a chronic ulcer

Sy   Chronic venous ulcer

Si   Ulcer with raised edge or any other atypical feature, local lymphadenopathy

Ix   Biopsy

Rx   Wide excision, skin graft may be necessary once margins are clear

Px   Long-term follow-up necessary as recurrence is possible

ANEURYSMS

TRUE ANEURYSM

P   Abnormal dilatation of an artery or the heart involving all layers of vessel wall

       May be saccular (protrudes from one side of vessel) or fusiform (generalized dilatation of vessel)

A   Many causes: atherosclerotic most common

Box 2.10 AETIOLOGY OF ANEURYSMS

- *Congenital weakness*: berry aneurysm in circle of Willis artery, Marfan's syndrome
- *Degenerative*: abdominal aortic aneurysm due to atherosclerosis
- *Trauma*: injury to vessel wall can cause weakness leading to true aneurysm formation
- *Infection*: bacterial arteritis
- *Inflammatory*: inflammatory process within arterial wall causes aneurysm formation (e.g. Kawasaki disease)

FALSE ANEURYSM (PSEUDOANEURYSM)

P   Haematoma containing liquid blood in contact with blood in arterial lumen

A   Due to trauma e.g. iatrogenic arterial puncture for angiography

Si   Pulsatile mass with history of trauma or arterial puncture (commonly in groin post-angioplasty)

Ix   Duplex USS

Rx   Direct pressure with USS probe, surgical repair of defect

ABDOMINAL AORTIC ANEURYSM (AAA)

A   Common in patients aged >60 years, more common in males

       May have a family history

P   May be atherosclerotic or inflammatory

       95 per cent are infrarenal

       Major risk is rupture; risk increases exponentially with aneurysm diameter

Sy   Back or loin pain; may be asymptomatic. Rupture causes severe pain and collapse

Si   Pulsatile mass, rupture causes hypovolaemic shock

Ix   USS, CT, rupture often clinical diagnosis requiring immediate surgery

Rx   Consider repair when diameter ≥5.5 cm

Regular USS surveillance if diameter <5 cm

Open repair with synthetic graft for elective and emergency cases, endovascular stent graft in selected patients

Modification of risk factors (BP/diabetic control) in patients with small aneurysms

Cx   Death, renal failure (if renal arteries involved), ischaemic bowel (inferior mesenteric involvement common), limb loss, paralysis, myocardial infarction, stroke, graft infection

Px   Elective operative mortality ~5 per cent

Rupture mortality ~75 per cent

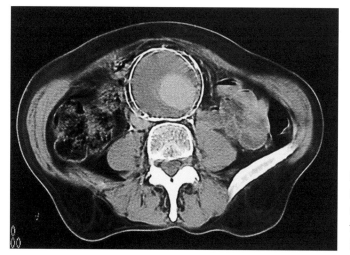

Figure 2.18 Calcified abdominal aortic aneurysm; the lumen of the aorta is surrounded by haematoma

AORTOENTERIC FISTULA

P   Abnormal communication between aorta and GI tract, usually duodenum/jejunum

A   Potentially life-threatening complication in patients who have had aortic surgery

Si   Brisk GI bleed with melaena, hypotension

Ix   Upper GI endoscopy, CT

Rx   Emergency surgery, graft replacement

Px   Poor

POPLITEAL ANEURYSM

A   Commonest peripheral aneurysm

Occurs in 10 per cent of patients with AAA, commonly bilateral

Sy   Often asymptomatic

Si   Pulsatile mass possibly bilateral, distal ischaemia following thrombosis or embolization

Ix   Duplex USS, angiography to assess distal vessels

Rx   Surgical bypass with ligation of popliteal artery

Cx   Thrombosis, distal embolization, rupture

Px   Good if treated electively

AORTIC DISSECTION

(P) Blood tracks through breach in intima creating parallel true and false lumens
Type A involves ascending aorta, Type B starts at origin of left subclavian artery

(A) Major risk factor is chronic hypertension

(Sy) Tearing chest pain radiating to back, hemiplegia, paraplegia, mesenteric or limb ischaemia

(Si) Shock, aortic regurgitation if aortic valve involved, unequal pulses or blood pressure unilaterally

(Ix) ECG, CXR shows widened mediastinum, CT, echocardiography

(Rx) *Type A:* surgical emergency requiring replacement of affected aorta using cardiopulmonary bypass
Type B: medical treatment of hypertension, may require surgical repair with graft if distal ischaemia occurs

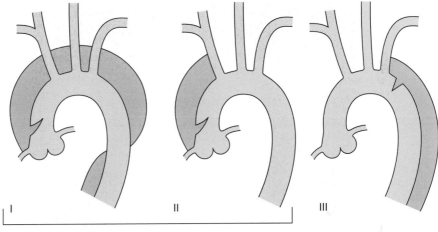

I   II   III

Type A   Type B

Figure 2.19 Classification of aortic dissection (reproduced with kind permission from Parker S, http://www.surgical-tutor.org.uk/default-home.htm?system/vascular/dissection.htm~right, accessed on 18 May 2006)

(Cx) Sudden death, stroke, mesenteric infarction, ischaemic limb, paralysis

(Px) Type A mortality high, Type B better prognosis

VENOUS REFLUX DISEASE

(P) Due to incompetence of venous valves
May occur in superficial, deep or perforating veins of legs
Superficial reflux may cause varicose veins

(A) Usually idiopathic, may be due to previous DVT (post-thrombotic limb) or raised venous pressure

(Sy) Leg swelling, aching, burning, cosmetic appearance

(Si) Deep and superficial reflux may cause leg swelling and skin changes including ulcers
Dilated tortuous superficial veins, palpable saphena varix, leg oedema, venous skin changes (venous eczema, venous flares, lipodermatosclerosis, atrophy blanche and ulceration)

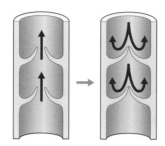

(a) Normal veins

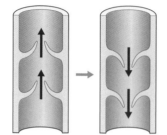

(b) Incompetent veins

Figure 2.20 Mechanism of venous reflux disease: (a) healthy venous valves; (b) varicose veins

 Venous duplex USS, venography

 Conservative: compression hosiery, injection sclerotherapy (high recurrence rate)
Surgery: only if deep venous incompetence is excluded. Ligation and stripping, endoluminal endothelial radiofrequency or laser ablation of incompetent veins accompanied by superficial avulsions. Ligation or endothelial ablation of incompetent perforator veins

Cx Venous ulcers cause disability and are costly to treat in the community

Px Recurrence after ligation and stripping remains common. Due to failure of surgical technique (e.g. failure to ligate all groin tributaries) or growth of neovascular tissue. Re-do surgery possible, but it has a higher complication rate than primary surgery

VENOUS THROMBOEMBOLISM

P Virchow's triad of predisposing conditions:
1. altered thrombotic tendency
2. altered blood flow
3. alteration to vessel wall

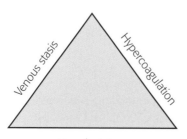

Figure 2.21 Virchow's triad

Surgery may induce all three

Peri-operative prevention is critical: early mobilization, compression hosiery, intermittent pneumatic pump, low-molecular weight heparin (LMWH, e.g. enoxaparin)

Box 2.11 COMMON CAUSES OF VENOUS THROMBOSIS

- Increasing age
- Thrombophilia
- Immobility
- Hormone replacement therapy (HRT)
- Surgery (especially pelvic/lower limb)
- Oral contraceptive pill (OCP)
- Malignancy
- Obesity

(Sy) Painful, swollen leg or arm

(Si) Variably swollen, tender, warm limb

(Ix) Duplex USS, D-dimer (excludes thrombosis if –ve), venography (rarely performed nowadays, but still considered 'gold standard')

(Rx) Anticoagulation, compression hosiery

(Cx) Pulmonary embolism – may be fatal, post-thrombotic limb

(Px) Good if treated promptly

LYMPHOEDEMA

(P) Failure of lymphatic drainage causes oedema

(A) Primary lymphoedema due to congenital lymphatic abnormality, onset may be at any age, more common in females

Secondary lymphoedema due to infection (e.g. recurrent cellulitis, filariasis), malignancy (e.g. axillary metastases from breast cancer), surgery (e.g. axillary clearance), radiotherapy or trauma causing lymphatic damage

(Sy) Swelling of limb, episodes of cellulitis

(Si) Swollen limb (foot typically affected), thick, scaly skin, lymphadenopathy if lymphoedema secondary to malignancy

(Ix) Lymphoscintigraphy compares uptake of isotope on each side

(Rx) *Conservative*: manual lymphatic drainage, pneumatic compression pump, compression hosiery

Surgery: severe cases only, removal of subcutaneous tissue and skin graft or lymphatic bypass, results often poor

(Cx) Recurrent cellulitis

(Px) Condition not curable, treatment aims to control symptoms

BREAST DISEASE

BENIGN BREAST DISEASE

LUMPS

Aetiology, treatment and prognosis are considered under individual headings

Ix   Triple assessment is the cornerstone of diagnosis:
1. clinical examination
2. radiological investigation (mammography, USS)
3. biopsy (fine needle aspiration for cytology, core biopsy for histology)

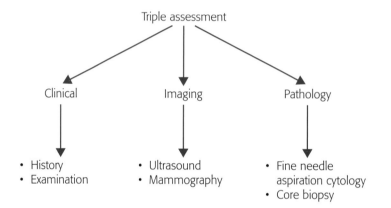

Figure 2.22 Triple assessment of breast lumps

FIBROADENOMA

P   Aberration of normal development, arise from whole lobule
A   Peak incidence in third decade, may occur at any age
Sy   Lump(s) usually painless
Si   Firm, highly mobile lump, may be multiple
Rx   *Conservative*: age <40 years, biopsy proven diagnosis
        Excision: age >40 years, size >4 cm or increasing, patient choice
Px   Usually remain unchanged, one-third resolve spontaneously

CYST

P   Enlarged, involuted lobule
A   Common in perimenopausal women
Sy   Lump(s) which may be painful
Si   Fluctuant or solid lump, may be tender, may be multiple
Rx   Aspiration, cytology of fluid only if bloody, biopsy of any residual lump after aspiration
Px   Commonly recur, slightly increased risk of breast cancer with cystic disease

PHYLLODES TUMOUR

P Uncommon fibroepithelial neoplasm
Majority are benign but may recur after excision
May be malignant but metastasis uncommon

S Firm lump, size may increase rapidly

Rx Wide excision, mastectomy for large tumours

DUCT PAPILLOMA

P Common benign neoplasm
Often occurs in subareolar ducts

S Single or multiple lump(s), nipple discharge which may be bloodstained

Rx Conservative or surgical excision of duct (microdochectomy)

FAT NECROSIS

A Often due to trauma

S History of trauma, firm lump, associated haematoma may be present
Clinically difficult to differentiate from carcinoma

Rx Conservative once diagnosis proven on biopsy

Px Usually resolves spontaneously

DUCT ECTASIA

P Normal changes in which ducts shorten and widen during breast involution in later life

S Lump, nipple discharge (may be bloody), nipple retraction (usually slit-like)

Rx Conservative, surgery for excessive discharge

LIPOMA

A Common benign neoplasm, may occur in breast

Ix May require excision to confirm diagnosis

BREAST PAIN (MASTALGIA)

A Very common, not associated with carcinoma

P Cyclical or non-cyclical

CYCLICAL BREAST PAIN

A Occurs in response to hormonal changes of menstrual cycle

Sy Pain from mid-cycle to menstruation, breast heaviness and lumpiness

Si Premenopausal woman, breast tenderness typically affects lateral half

Rx Reassurance, gamolenic acid (evening primrose oil – slow response, few side-effects), danazol and bromocriptine (side-effects common)

NON-CYCLICAL BREAST PAIN

A Pain may arise in the breast or chest wall
Usually postmenopausal women

Sy Pain may be continuous or intermittent

Ix Exclude referred pain e.g. arthritis of chest wall, lung disease

Rx Reassurance, simple measures e.g. ensure correctly fitted bra, non-steroidal anti-inflammatory medications, gamolenic acid, surgery not indicated

INFECTION

LACTATING

P *Staphylococcus aureus* most common pathogen

Sy Pain, tenderness, swelling, redness

Si Pyrexia, erythema, tenderness, fluctuance indicates abscess

Rx Antibiotics, aspiration or incision and drainage of abscess, continue breast feeding

NON-LACTATING

P Caused by aerobic and anaerobic bacteria

A Smoking is a risk factor

Sy Pain, tenderness, redness, may have lump

Si Pyrexia, erythema, tenderness, inflammatory mass or abscess may occur

Rx Antibiotics, aspiration or incision and drainage of abscess, investigation of any residual lump after treatment

Cx Mammary duct fistula requires surgical excision

GYNAECOMASTIA

P Benign breast tissue growth in males (carcinoma must be excluded)

A Occurs at any age, common in elderly and at puberty

Box 2.12 CAUSES OF GYNAECOMASTIA

- Idiopathic
- Digoxin
- Cimetidine
- Spironolactone
- Cannabis
- Cirrhosis
- Renal failure
- Testicular tumours

S Unilateral or bilateral soft, diffuse lump, may be painful

Ix Mammography if any suspicious signs (1 per cent of all breast cancer occurs in males)

Rx *Conservative*: withdrawal of drugs, danazol, tamoxifen
Surgery: occasionally indicated

Px Usually responds to conservative treatment

MALIGNANT BREAST DISEASE

DUCTAL CARCINOMA *IN SITU* (DCIS)

P Carcinoma which has not penetrated basement membrane
DCIS most common form of breast carcinoma *in situ*
Graded as low- to high-grade lesions on histology

(S) Lump, nipple discharge, asymptomatic screening detected

(Ix) Triple assessment (see p. 144)

(Rx) According to size of lesion, wide local excision (WLE) and radiotherapy, mastectomy, consider tamoxifen

(Px) Follow up with regular mammography to detect recurrence

Risk of progression to invasive carcinoma, highest risk for high-grade DCIS

LOBULAR CARCINOMA *IN SITU*

(A) Rare condition

(Rx) Treatment by observation, tamoxifen or bilateral mastectomy ($\uparrow$ risk of carcinoma in contralateral breast)

(Px) Risk of progression to invasive carcinoma

INVASIVE CARCINOMA

(A) Most common cancer in females

Lifetime risk approximately 1 in 10 (increasing)

Occurs at any age, rare under 30 years

Box 2.13 RISK FACTORS FOR BREAST CANCER

- Female sex (1 per cent of cancers in males)
- Age
- Family history: genes include *BRCA1* and *BRCA2*
- Early menarche, late menopause
- Nulliparity, higher age at first pregnancy
- Higher socioeconomic group
- HRT: small effect

Assessment and treatment should be in a specialist breast unit

Treatment is multimodality involving surgery, radiotherapy and chemotherapy

Diagnosis and assessment

- Presentation with palpable lump or screening-detected abnormality
- Triple assessment of any breast lump: clinical examination, radiological investigation (mammography/ultrasound) and biopsy
- Histological grading 1, 2 or 3 according to differentiation
- TNM (tumour, node, metastasis) staging according to tumour size, lymph node involvement and metastases
- Staging involves examination, radiological investigation (e.g. CXR, abdominal USS or CT) and surgery

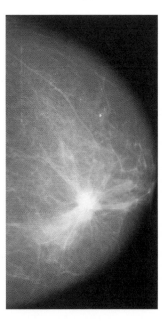

Figure 2.23 Breast carcinoma: spiculated mass on mammography

Breast surgery

- According to size of tumour and size of breast
- Breast-conserving surgery involves WLE followed by radiotherapy
- Clear resection margins are important
- Mastectomy if tumour too large for breast-conserving surgery or for patient choice
- Reconstructive surgery can be simultaneous with mastectomy or delayed
- Reconstruction is by myocutaneous flap based on the latissimus dorsi or rectus abdominis

Axillary surgery

- Performed for almost all invasive cancers
  Axillary clearance can be level 2 (includes nodes lateral and deep to the pectoralis minor) or level 3 (also includes apical nodes)
- For smaller tumours axillary node sampling or sentinel node biopsy are options
- Sampling requires at least four random nodes for examination
- Positive node sampling or biopsy requires further axillary treatment by clearance or radiotherapy
- Axillary clearance and radiotherapy carry risk of arm lymphoedema

---

INFORMATION BOX: SENTINEL NODE BIOPSY

Sentinel node biopsy involves identification of the first node draining the tumour by injecting radioactive isotope and coloured dye. Sampling this node indicates whether lymphatic spread has occurred, and saves some women the need for extensive axillary surgery.

Adjuvant therapy

- Tamoxifen or anastrozole (Arimidex, AstraZeneca) for oestrogen receptor-positive tumours
- Cytotoxic chemotherapy for patients at high risk of recurrence e.g. node-positive disease
- Radiotherapy to the breast following breast-conserving surgery
- Radiotherapy to the chest wall following mastectomy in those at high risk of recurrence
- Radiotherapy to axilla in selected cases e.g. positive node sample

Paget's disease of the nipple

- **(P)** Eczematous skin change to the nipple due to underlying malignancy
- **(Si)** May have associated lump
- **(Ix)** Triple assessment (see p. 144) including incisional skin biopsy
- **(Rx)** Mastectomy and axillary clearance if separate mass present
  WLE and radiotherapy possible if mass lies behind nipple

SCREENING

- Self-examination
- Two-view mammography offered every three years to UK women aged 50 to 64 years
- After age of 64 years women can self-refer for mammograms if they wish
- Suspicious mammographic sign prompts recall
- Screen-detected cancers generally smaller and lower grade than symptomatic lesions
- Drawbacks include cost and potential psychological morbidity of false positives

ENDOCRINE SURGERY

THYROID GLAND

CONGENITAL ANOMALIES

Box 2.14 CONGENITAL THYROID ABNORMALITIES

- *Lingual thyroid*
  - failure of descent of part or all of the thyroid into the neck
  - presents with a lump at the back of the tongue
- *Thyroglossal cyst*:
  - thyroglossal duct sometimes remains along the tract of the thyroid descent from the tongue to the neck
  - cyst may develop in a persistent duct
  - presents with a midline neck lump which moves up on protrusion of the tongue
  - treatment is surgical excision of the lump and duct remnant, may require excision of part of the hyoid bone
- *Thyroglossal fistula*
  - patent thyroglossal duct remnant opening onto the skin
  - presents with a fluid discharge from fistula
  - treatment is surgical excision of fistula, duct remnant and part of the hyoid bone

---

THYROTOXICOSIS (GRAVES' DISEASE)

This is covered in detail on p. 68.

Rx   Thyroidectomy is often needed for disease refractory to medical therapy

Cx   See Box 2.15

Box 2.15 COMPLICATIONS OF THYROIDECTOMY

- Haemorrhage causing airway compression
- Recurrent laryngeal nerve injury (hoarse voice)
- Thyroid crisis
- Injury to parathyroids (hypoparathyroidism + hypocalcaemia)
- Hypothyroidism

Px   Good after surgery, relapse frequent with medical therapy

GOITRE

P   Defined as enlargement of the thyroid gland

A   See Box 2.16

Box 2.16 CAUSES OF GOITRE

- *Physiological*:
  - due to puberty, pregnancy or iodine deficiency
  - iodine replacement may be required
- *Nodular*:
  - commonest cause in Western world
  - gland diffusely enlarged and irregular
  - patient usually euthyroid but may be thyrotoxic if dominant nodule is overactive
  - treatment indicated for thyrotoxicosis, compression of adjacent structures or suspicion of malignant change
- *Toxic goitre*:
  - Graves' disease
- *Hashimoto's disease*:
  - antithyroid autoantibodies produced
  - gland diffusely enlarged
  - patient usually hypothyroid
  - treatment with thyroxine
- *de Quervain's thyroiditis*:
  - gland inflammation due to viral infection
  - thyroid enlarged and tender
  - classically causes hyper- and then hypothyroidism
  - usually resolves spontaneously
- *Riedel's thyroiditis*:
  - gland infiltration with scar tissue
  - biopsy to differentiate from carcinoma
  - usually causes hypothyroidism
  - conservative treatment, thyroxine may be required

Ix TFT, thyroid antibodies, radio-isotope scan, USS, FNA for cytology

Rx See under individual causes

BENIGN NEOPLASMS

- Thyroid cysts may be aspirated, may require excision as recurrence is common
- Follicular adenoma can only be differentiated from carcinoma on histology, excision is therefore required
- Dominant nodule in nodular goitre: no treatment required but may need excision to prove diagnosis

THYROID CANCER

See Box 2.17

Box 2.17 SUBTYPES OF THYROID CANCER

- *Papillary carcinoma*:
    commonest
    age 10–40 years, ♀ > ♂
    slow growing, spread to lymph nodes occurs late
- *Follicular carcinoma*:
    age 40–60 years, ♀ > ♂
    may arise in nodular goitre
    spread is by blood
- *Medullary carcinoma*:
    any age, ♀ = ♂
    arises in parafollicular C cells and secretes calcitonin
    associated with multiple endocrine neoplasia
- *Anaplastic carcinoma*:
    elderly patients, ♀ > ♂
    rapid growth
    early local invasion and spread by lymphatics
- *Lymphoma*:
    uncommon

Sy Lump, sometimes pain, dysphagia, hoarse voice
Si Lump, sometimes cervical lymphadenopathy
Ix TFT, radio-isotope scan, USS, fine needle aspiration (FNA)
Rx *Papillary*:
- thyroid lobectomy or total thyroidectomy
- block dissection of involved nodes
- long-term thyroxine to suppress remaining thyroid
Follicular:
- thyroid lobectomy or total thyroidectomy
- block dissection of involved nodes
- long-term thyroxine replacement
- radioactive iodine may be used to supplement surgery or for secondary disease
Medullary:
- total thyroidectomy
- block dissection of involved nodes
- calcitonin used as marker for recurrence
Anaplastic:
- frequently inoperable
- palliative radiotherapy often given
Px Good for papillary, follicular and medullary cancer, very poor for anaplastic carcinoma

OTHER NECK LUMPS

- *Lymph node*: common, reactive or due to tumour deposit, investigation for associated malignancy e.g. head and neck, lymphoma
- *Cystic hygroma*: congenital cystic mass developing in remnant of jugular lymph sac, usually seen in children, transilluminates, treatment by surgical excision

- *Branchial cyst*: remnant of branchial arch, lies anterior and deep to sternocleidomastoid, may form abscess, treatment by surgical excision
- *Carotid body tumour*: tumour of chemoreceptor cells, slow growing, may metastasize late, may be pulsatile, treatment surgical or conservative (in the elderly)
- *Carotid aneurysm*: pulsatile, expansile mass

MISCELLANEOUS

CARCINOID TUMOUR

(P) Tumour arising from amine precursor uptake and decarboxylation (APUD) cells
Secretes 5-hydroxytryptamine (5-HT)
May occur anywhere in the gastrointestinal tract or lung
Site: appendix 35 per cent, ileum 28 per cent, rectum 13 per cent and bronchi 13 per cent

(A) Most common neuroendocrine tumour (incidence 2–7 per million)
♀ = ♂, tends to occur in those aged over 30 years

(S) *Carcinoid tumour*: few initially. May present as appendicitis or obstruction
Carcinoid syndrome: hepatomegaly, profuse colicky diarrhoea, cutaneous flushing, abdominal pain, right-sided cardiac valve disease and bronchoconstriction

(Ix) *Urine*: 24-h urine collection for 5-hydroxyindoleacetic acid (5-HIAA) which is a metabolite of 5-HT
Imaging: CT/USS of liver. MIBG (metaiodobenzylguanidine) nuclear medicine scan to localize primary tumour

(Rx) Resection of tumour and possibly liver secondaries, chemotherapy, sometimes only symptomatic treatment with 5-HT antagonists, somatostatin analogues

(Px) Slow-growing tumour, patients commonly survive many years
Median survival ~ 5–8 years

MULTIPLE ENDOCRINE NEOPLASIA (MEN)

(P) Rare syndromes involving endocrine adenomas or adenocarcinomas
MEN 1:
  – autosomal dominant inheritance
  – parathyroid tumour
  – pancreatic islet cell tumour
  – pituitary tumour
MEN 2a:
  – autosomal dominant inheritance
  – thyroid medullary carcinoma
  – phaeochromocytoma
  – parathyroid tumour
MEN 2b:
  – thyroid medullary carcinoma
  – phaeochromocytoma
  – mucocutaneous ganglioneuromas

BURNS

A Thermal, electrical, chemical or irradiation
P Tissue damage related to temperature and duration of burn
Assessment: airway, breathing, circulation (ABC)
Use the Wallace 'rule of nines' chart (see Box 2.18 and Figure 2.24)

Box 2.18 THE WALLACE 'RULE OF NINES'

●	Head and neck	9%
●	Each arm	9%
●	Anterior trunk	18%
●	Posterior trunk	18%
●	Each leg	18%
●	Perineum	1%
●	Total	100%

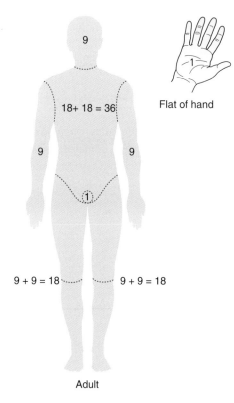

Figure 2.24 Wallace 'rule of nines' chart

Lund and Browder charts are more accurate and take account of patient age
Classified as full or partial thickness depending on how much epithelium has been lost

Table 2.3 Differentiation of full- and partial-thickness burns

Full thickness	Partial thickness
May be painless	Painful
Sloughy	Reddened, may blister
Heals by granulation tissue and scarring	Heals by growth of new epithelium

Rx

A:
- may require intubation

B:
- 100 per cent O_2
- measure carboxyhaemoglobin if carbon monoxide poisoning suspected. May require hyperbaric oxygen
- may require escharotomy if thoracic burns limit chest movement

C:
- *Fluid replacement:* according to formula such as Muir and Barclay: give (weight in kg × per cent burn × 0.5) mls of colloid over each time period (4, 4, 4, 6, 6 and 12 h)
- *Analgesia:* opiates often required
- *Escharotomy:* full-thickness circumferential burns to limb or thorax may restrict blood flow or breathing. Performed to save life or limb

Refer to specialist burns unit if burns >10 per cent in children or elderly and >20 per cent at other ages

FLUID BALANCE

70KG MAN

- 60 per cent water = 42 L
- Extracellular fluid (ECF) = 14 L
  - plasma: 3 L
  - interstitial fluid: 11 L
  - transcellular fluid: small amount
- Intracellular fluid (ICF) = 28 L
- Transcellular fluid includes cerebrospinal, intraocular, pericardial, pleural and peritoneal fluid

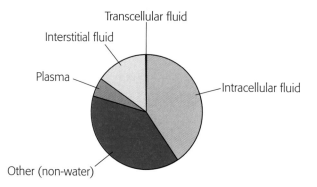

Figure 2.25 Pie chart showing proportions of fluid in an adult

NORMAL DAILY REQUIREMENT

- *Replacement of*:
  - insensible loss e.g. faeces, lungs – 500 mL
  - urine – 1000 mL
  - insensible loss from skin – 500–2000 mL
- *Basic regime each 24 h*:
  - 3000 mL water
  - 100 mmol sodium
  - 60 mmol potassium
- *This can be achieved with*:
  - 1000 mL normal saline
  - 2000 mL 5 per cent dextrose
  - 20 mmol potassium with each 1000 mL of fluid

ASSESSMENT OF FLUID STATUS

- Thirst
- Skin turgor, tongue, mucous membranes
- Pulse, blood pressure, jugular venous pressure (JVP)
- Urine output (should be at least 0.5 mL/kg/h)

- Input/output charts with overall 24-h fluid balance
- Blood urea and electrolyte measurement
- Central venous pressure: absolute value less useful than trend following intravenous fluid administration
- Fluid replacement: maintenance fluids + replacement of abnormal losses such as vomit, blood and third space fluid e.g. in pancreatitis

Table 2.4 Types of intravenous fluid

Crystalloid	Colloid
Electrolytes in solution in water	Contain high-molecular weight particles
Distribute rapidly through ECF volume	Remain in circulation and exert oncotic pressure, drawing interstitial fluid into plasma
Include normal saline, Hartmann's solution, 5% dextrose	Include blood, Haemaccel (Syner-Med), Gelofusine (Braun)

PARENTERAL NUTRITION

- Intravenous nutrition
- Given until enteral feeding is possible
- *Indications*:
  - enteral feeding not possible for >4 days
  - multiple injuries
  - malabsorption
  - intestinal fistulae
- Administered in co-operation with dietitian/nutritionist
- Usually administered via central vein as solutions are hypertonic and damage smaller veins
- *Composition*:
  - carbohydrate and lipid provide calories
  - protein
  - trace elements and vitamins
- *Monitoring*:
  - daily weight
  - blood tests for electrolytes and albumin

NEUROSURGERY

HEAD INJURY

 Common at all ages

May lead to skull fractures and brain injuries

Skull fractures:
– facial bones
– base of skull
– skull vault

Brain injuries: primary due to direct trauma
– Coup: at site of impact
– Contre-coup: brain impacts skull on opposite side to that of trauma
– Shear: causes diffuse axonal injury

Secondary brain injury due to delayed effects of injury e.g. hypoxia, intracranial haemorrhage

Cerebral perfusion depends on cerebral perfusion pressure = blood pressure – intracranial pressure (ICP)

Head injury can cause ↑ICP which ↓ cerebral perfusion pressure

Classification:
– minor (Glasgow Coma Score (GCS) 13–15)
– moderate (GCS 9–12)
– severe (GCS <9)

INFORMATION BOX: GLASGOW COMA SCORE

- Standardized means of assessing and describing conscious level
- Possible score from 3 to 15
- GCS ≤ 8 is defined as coma (see Table 2.5)

 Airway with cervical spine immobilization

Breathing

Circulation

Specialist treatment depends on extent and type of injuries and is discussed later

Table 2.5 Glasgow Coma Scale

Observation	Score
Eye opening	
Spontaneous	4
To speech	3
To pain	2
None	1
Best verbal response	
Orientated	5
Confused	4
Inappropriate words	3
Incomprehensible sounds	2
None	1
Best motor response	
Obeys commands	6
Localizes to pain	5
Withdraws from pain	4
Abnormal flexion	3
Extension	2
None	1
Total	/15

INTRACRANIAL HAEMORRHAGE

SUBARACHNOID HAEMORRHAGE

P Traumatic or secondary to leaking aneurysm

Sy Sudden-onset headache, 'the worst headache of my life, doctor'

Si Neck stiffness, photophobia

Ix CT, cerebral angiography

Rx *Conservative*
Surgery: clipping or embolization of aneurysm

SUBDURAL HAEMORRHAGE

P Tear of venous bridging veins between cortex and venous sinuses

A Acute due to severe head injury
Chronic common in alcoholics and elderly, often due to minor head injury, especially if anticoagulated

S Headache, weakness, numbness, slurred speech, nausea/vomiting, lethargy, seizures

Ix CT

Rx Surgical evacuation of haematoma

Px Related to severity of head injury

EXTRADURAL HAEMORRHAGE

P   Trauma causes damage to extradural vessel

Si ICP rises causing decreasing GCS

Compression of 3rd cranial nerve (false localizing sign) causes ipsilateral pupil dilatation

Rx Immediate surgical decompression to prevent death

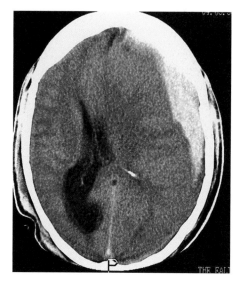

Figure 2.26 CT brain scan: subdural haemorrhage

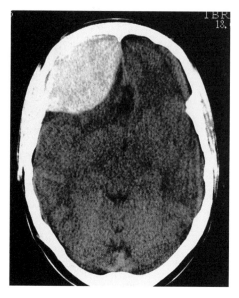

Figure 2.27 CT brain scan: extradural haemorrhage

NEUROLOGICAL TUMOURS

GLIOMA

A   Arise from glial cells in the brain

P   Divided into astrocytomas (most common), medulloblastomas, ependymomas and oligodendrogliomas according to the cell type of origin

Rx Surgical excision where possible

Palliative treatment is often the only option and includes surgery, chemotherapy and radiotherapy

MENINGIOMA

A   Arise from arachnoid cells in the meninges

P   Usually benign and slow growing

Rx Surgical excision

ACOUSTIC NEUROMA

A   Arise from Schwann cells of cranial nerve 8 (associated with neurofibromatosis)

P   Presses on 5th, 7th, 9th, 10th and 12th cranial nerves as tumour expands

Sy Unilateral deafness, facial numbness and weakness

Rx Surgical excision but risks nerve damage

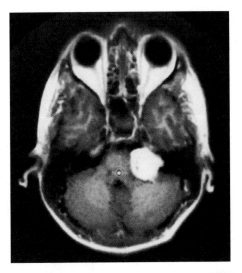

Figure 2.28 Acoustic neuroma: mass of increased signal at the cerebellopontine angle

PITUITARY TUMOURS

 Usually adenomas
May cause endocrine abnormalities e.g. hypopituitarism, Cushing's syndrome

(Si) May compress optic chiasm causing bitemporal hemianopia

(Rx) Surgical excision or hormonal manipulation

LYMPHOMA

(A) Uncommon, occurs with increased frequency in AIDS

(Rx) Radiotherapy

(Px) Poor, survival often <1 year

METASTASES

(A) Common

(P) Principally from primaries in breast, lung, kidney and malignant melanoma

(Rx) Supportive, steroids

OTHER CNS DISORDERS

SPINAL CORD COMPRESSION

 Compression of the spinal cord is an emergency

(A) Vertebral metastases, abscess, disc prolapse, cord tumour, trauma

(Sy) Sudden-onset leg weakness, leg pain, sensory loss, painless urinary retention

(Si) Sensory level, motor weakness, hyperreflexia

(Ix) MRI

(Rx) *Metastases*: steroids, radiotherapy, surgical decompression
Abscess: drainage, antibiotics
Disc prolapse: surgical decompression

(Cx) Paralysis, neurogenic bladder

(Px) Depends on cause. Best chance of recovery with early treatment

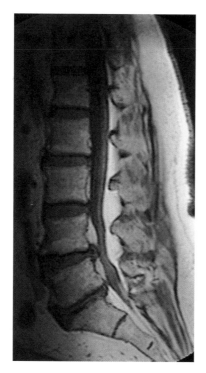

Figure 2.29 Lumbar disc prolapse: the MRI scan shows a L4/5 disc protrusion extending up to the theca

CAUDA EQUINA SYNDROME

(A) Compression of the cauda equina has the same causes as cord compression
(S) Commonly causes back pain, bladder and bowel sphincter dysfunction
Leg weakness occurs together with absent reflexes
(Rx) Treatment varies with cause as for cord compression

HYDROCEPHALUS

(P) Raised cerebrospinal fluid (CSF) pressure in the ventricular system of the brain
(A) Obstruction of the normal production, circulation and reabsorption pathway of CSF within the ventricles
May be congenital or acquired

INFORMATION BOX: HYDROCEPHALUS

- *Non-communicating hydrocephalus* is due to obstruction of CSF flow from the brain to the subarachnoid space – may be due to congenital malformation or development of a tumour.
- *Communicating hydrocephalus* is due to failure of CSF reabsorption from the subarachnoid space – may be due to congenital abnormality in arachnoid villi, meningitis or subarachnoid haemorrhage.

(Rx) Treatment is by relief of pressure with a shunt or resection of any obstructing lesion

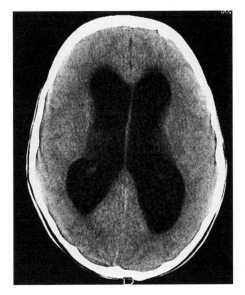

Figure 2.30 Hydrocephalus: dilatation of the ventricles without enlargement of the sulci

PERIPHERAL NERVOUS SYSTEM DISORDERS

SCIATICA

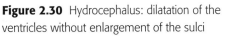 Sciatic nerve originates from L4–5 and S1–3 nerve roots
Compression of nerve root by prolapsed intervertebral disc causes leg pain

Sy Pain typically shoots down leg to below knee

Si Limited straight leg raise due to pain, decreased sensation over relevant dermatome, muscle weakness (weak hallux extension in L5 compression, foot plantar flexion in S1)

Ix MRI

Rx Conservative treatment usually effective, surgical discectomy in selected cases

Px Complete resolution may take months

MERALGIA PARAESTHETICA

P Compression of the lateral cutaneous nerve of the thigh
Occurs as nerve exits beneath inguinal ligament

A Caused by obesity and extrinsic compression from overly tight belts/clothing

S Causes pain and altered sensation over anterior and lateral part of thigh which is relieved by hip flexion

Rx *Conservative:* weight loss, loose clothing
Surgery: decompression may be effective in difficult cases

CARPAL TUNNEL SYNDROME

 Compression of the median nerve within the carpal tunnel (deep to the flexor retinaculum)

 Associated with pregnancy, rheumatoid arthritis, acromegaly, hypothyroidism

 Pain and paraesthesia in radial three digits
Wasting of thenar muscles

Conservative: splinting
Surgery: steroid injection, surgical carpal tunnel decompression (division of flexor retinaculum)

BRACHIAL PLEXUS LESIONS

- *Upper trunk lesion: Erb's palsy*
  - occurs with forced contralateral neck abduction
  - C5 and 6 nerve roots injured
  - arm internally rotated with extended elbow (waiter's tip position)
  - decreased sensation over C5 and 6 dermatomes
- *T1 lesion: Klumpke's palsy*
  - occurs with shoulder dislocation or cervical rib
  - wasting of intrinsic muscles of hand
  - decreased sensation over T1 dermatome

RADIAL NERVE LESIONS

A Commonly injured in fractures of spiral groove of humerus
Si Wrist drop
Decreased sensation over dorsum of first webspace

ULNAR NERVE LESIONS

A Commonly injured in fractures around elbow and lacerations
Si Causes clawing of the 4th and 5th digits (*main en griffe*)
Decreased sensation over ulnar one-and-a-half digits

CHAPTER 3

Orthopaedics

Julian Leong

FRACTURE

P A fracture is a break in the continuity of the cortex of a bone

CLASSIFICATIONS

- Closed (simple) versus open (compound):
  - open fractures are associated with an break in the skin, therefore making the fracture site potentially 'dirty'
  - Gustilo–Anderson classification Type I–III according to extent of soft tissue damage

Table 3.1 Gustilo–Anderson classification of open fractures

Grade	Characteristics
Type I	Clean wound smaller than 1 cm in diameter, simple fracture pattern, no skin crushing
Type II	A laceration larger than 1 cm but without significant soft tissue crushing, including no flaps, degloving or contusion
Type III	An open segmental fracture or a single fracture with extensive soft tissue injury. Also included are injuries older than 8 h

- *Linear*: transverse, oblique and spiral
- *Comminuted*: more than two fragments
- Fractures associated with the epiphysis of the bone (where growth occurs) were classified by Salter–Harris: five types of fractures associated with physeal injuries in immature bone

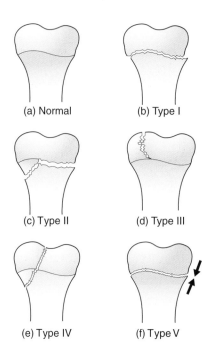

Figure 3.1 Salter Harris classification of epiphyseal injuries (a) Normal; (b) Type I: epiphyseal slip only; (c) Type II: fracture through the epiphyseal plate with a triangle of shaft attached; (d) Type III: fracture through the epiphysis extending into the epiphyseal plate; (e) Type IV: fracture of the epiphysis, crossing the epiphyseal plate; (f) Type V: damage to the epiphyseal plate

COMPLICATIONS

IMMEDIATE (MINUTES TO HOURS)

- Pain
- Nerve, blood vessel, skin and muscle damage
- Fat embolism
- Visceral damage (pneumothorax in rib fracture, etc.)
- Insufficient skin coverage (open fracture)

EARLY (HOURS TO DAYS)

- Compartment syndrome (see p. 167)
- Immobility
- Wound infection
- Deep venous thrombosis and pulmonary embolism

LATE (WEEKS TO MONTHS)

- Stiffness
- Sudek's atrophy (complex regional pain syndrome/regional sympathetic dystrophy/reflex osteodystrophy)
- Malunion, delayed union, non-union
- Pseudoarthritis
- Secondary osteoarthritis (intra-articular fracture)
- Chronic osteomyelitis (open fracture)

PRINCIPLES OF FRACTURE MANAGEMENT

- Fractures can vary in severity from insignificant occurrences not warranting any treatment to life- or limb-threatening episodes
- For serious/multiple fractures use advanced trauma life support (ATLS) guidelines (ABC – airway, breathing, circulation)
- The history should reveal the mechanism of injury, premorbid conditions and fitness for surgery
- *Examination*: general and specific to reveal any occult injuries
- *Investigations*: baseline pre-operative investigations and radiographs for suspected fracture sites

GENERAL TREATMENT

- Analgesia,
- Deep vein thrombosis (DVT) prophylaxis with low-molecular weight heparin (LMWH), for hip fractures or anticipated immobilization and anti-embolism stockings (TEDS)
- Treat other injuries

FRACTURE-SPECIFIC TREATMENT

1. *Reduce*:
   - for displaced fractures
2. *Hold*:
- Non-operative:
   - *simple splinting*: neighbouring strap (e.g. mid-shaft metacarpal fractures)
   - *plaster of Paris (POP)*: cheap, effective, bulky (relative stability)
   - *Fibreglass cast*: lighter and less bulky than POP
- Operative:
   - *internal fixation*: Kirschner wire (K wire); screws and plate; intramedullary device
   - *external fixation*: uniplanar or circular wire (e.g. Ilizarov frame)
3. *Rehabilitate*:
   - physiotherapy, walking aid, occupational therapy, social worker

OTHER EMERGENCY TREATMENTS

- Almost always need to precede fracture treatment
- *Dislocation*: reduction – closed (without cutting the skin) if possible
- *Open fracture*: tetanus immunization update, broad-spectrum antibiotics, urgent debridement and washout
- *Compartment syndrome*: emergency fasciotomy
- *Vascular compromise*: angiography ± vascular repair

COMPARTMENT SYNDROME

 Increased pressure in a closed fascial compartment, usually secondary to injury

Results in venous stasis and leakage of capillary exudates inside the compartment
This leads to a vicious circle and further increases the compartmental pressure preventing blood flow into the compartment
Ultimately, irreversible muscle necrosis occurs if treatment is not performed in time

Pain out of proportion to the injury
Pain in passive stretch of the muscular compartment
Paraesthesiae and pulselessness are late signs

Rx If suspected: emergency fasciotomy (division of fascia to relieve pressure) before late signs occur

COMMON TRAUMA

UPPER LIMB

PROXIMAL HUMERUS

 Often occurs in the elderly, ♀:♂ 2:1
Fall from standing height, road traffic accident

P Can be comminuted (Neer's classification)

Rx Usually treated conservatively in collar-and-cuff, with good results
Physiotherapy
Comminuted fractures may need open reduction and internal fixation (ORIF) or shoulder hemiarthroplasty

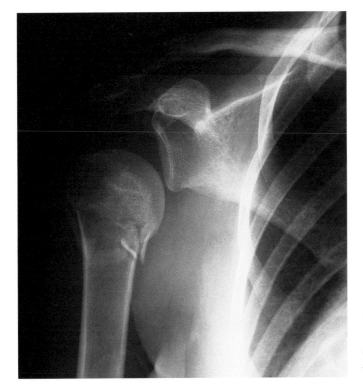

Figure 3.2 Humeral neck fracture with downward subluxation of the humeral head

SHOULDER DISLOCATION

P Most commonly anterior and inferior dislocation

A First episodes are often traumatic
Posterior dislocation can occur in an epileptic fit

 Pain, decreased movement

 Loss of deltoid contour, arm held internally rotated and adducted
Must examine and document axillary nerve function (sensation to the regimental arm badge area) before attempting reduction

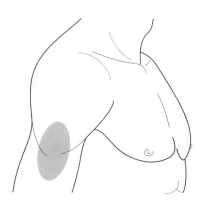

Figure 3.3 Region of the arm supplied by the axillary nerve

 X-rays: anteroposterior (AP) and axial (or Y view)

Reduction (emergency – sedated or under anaesthesia)

Consent

Modified Kocher's technique

Must re-examine the axillary nerve post-reduction

Immobilize with a broad arm sling

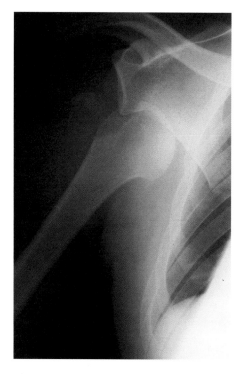

Figure 3.4 Anterior dislocation of the shoulder

ROTATOR CUFF DISORDERS

Rotator cuff consists of:

- *insertion into the greater tuberosity:* supraspinatus (abduction), infraspinatus (external rotation), teres minor (external rotation)
- *insertion into the lesser tuberosity:* subscapularis (internal rotation)
- **(P)** Degenerative changes, trauma and attempted healing resulting in tendonitis (acute or chronic) ± tears (complete or partial)

Acute calcifying tendonitis

- **(P)** Involves the supraspinatus tendon
- **(A)** Presents with acutely painful shoulder after vigorous activity
- **(Ix)** X-ray often shows calcification in the tendon
- **(Rx)** Usually resolves with non-operative treatment

Chronic tendonitis

- **(P)** Otherwise known as impingement syndrome (as the tendon is compressed against the coracoacromial arch) or painful arc syndrome
- **(A)** Middle-aged patients with pain in active shoulder abduction between 60° and 120°
- **(Ix)** MRI or USS
- **(Rx)** *Non-operative:* physiotherapy, NSAIDs, and joint injection
  Operative: subacromial decompression ± tendon repair

Tendon tears

- **(P)** Complete tears abolish active movement of the particular muscle and partial tears present as pain and weakness.

BICEPS TENDON RUPTURE

- **(P)** Similar to rotator cuff disorders, and presents with 'Popeye' sign (biceps muscle retracting up the upper arm, creating a bulge)

FROZEN SHOULDER (ADHESIVE CAPSULITIS)

- **(A)** Middle-aged patient with severe pain after often trivial trauma
- **(Si)** Loss of range of movement in active and passive movement (especially external rotation)
- **(Ix)** X-ray may show osteoporosis
- **(Rx)** Analgesia, NSAIDs, physiotherapy ± manipulation under anaesthesia

DISTAL RADIUS

- *Extra-articular:*
  - Colles' fracture – shortened, dorsal displacement, dorsal angulation of the distal fragment
  - Smith's fracture – shortened, volar displacement, volar angulation of the distal fragment

(a)

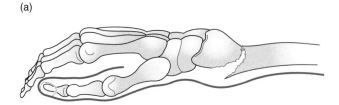

(b)

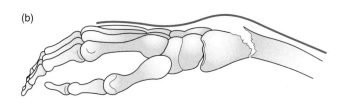

Figure 3.5 (a) extension fracture of the radius (Colles' fracture); (b) flexion fracture of the radius (Smith's fracture);

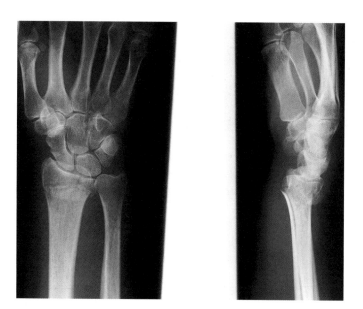

Figure 3.6 Colles' fracture: a fracture of the distal radius with posterior displacement of the distal fragment, best seen on the lateral projection

- *Intra-articular*:
    - Barton's fracture: fracture subluxation of the distal radius
    - Galeazzi fracture: distal radial fracture with dislocation of the distal radio-ulnar joint
    - Monteggia fracture: proximal ulnar fracture with dislocation of the radial head

SCAPHOID FRACTURE

Sy Pain and swelling in the wrist after falling on an outstretched hand

Si Tenderness at anatomical snuff box and telescoping the thumb

Ix AP and lateral radiographs of the hand and wrist

Scaphoid views (10 day post-injury ± immediate post-injury)

If diagnosis is uncertain (common), repeat clinical and radiological examination without the plaster 10 days post-injury

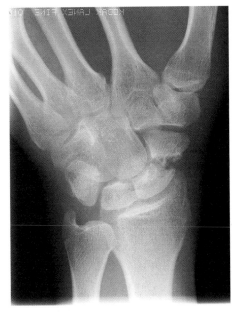

Figure 3.7 Non-union of a scaphoid fracture

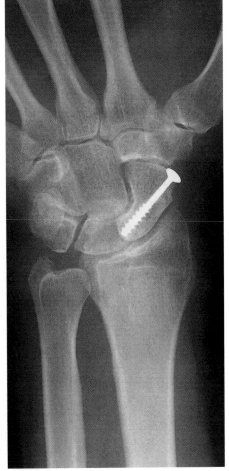

Figure 3.8 Internal fixation of a scaphoid fracture

Rx All suspected fractures (tender at the anatomical snuff box) are initially treated with a scaphoid plaster.
Internal fixation with Herbert screw – for fracture non-union or displaced fractures

Cx Blood supply of the scaphoid bone enters distally; hence fracture of the waist of the scaphoid bone can result in avascular necrosis of the proximal part

BENNETT'S FRACTURE

A Most common thumb injury

P Intra-articular fracture dislocation of the first metacarpal bone

Rx Often needs fixation with either K-wires or screws

BOXER'S FRACTURE

(A) Often associated with punching

(P) Fracture of the neck of the 5th metacarpal bone

(Rx) If clinically no rotational deformity, treat with neighbour strapping (buddy strap)

LOWER LIMB

FRACTURED NECK OF FEMUR

(A) 50 000 admissions per year in the over 60 age group in England

Patients often elderly and osteoporotic, with associated medical problems

(Sy) Pain in the hip after fall, unable to weight-bear

(Si) Affected side with shortened and externally rotated leg

(Ix) AP pelvic X-ray and lateral affected hip (full length femur if pathological fracture suspected)

Box 3.1 CLASSIFICATION OF FRACTURES OF THE FEMORAL NECK

- *Intracapsular fracture*:
  - subcapital, transcervical – classified by Garden I–IV relating to amount of displacement of fragments
- *Extracapsular fracture*:
  - basi-cervical
  - intertrochanteric, subtrochanteric – strictly not neck of femur

---

(Rx) *Non operative*: rare, unless operative mortality precludes operation

Internal fixation:
- Garden I–II intracapsular fracture, young patient (cannulated screws) or any patient with extracapsular fracture (dynamic hip screw or intra-medullary device)
- older patient with Garden III–IV intracapsular fracture (higher risk of avascular necrosis of the femoral head): hemiarthroplasty (uncemented Austin Moore or cemented bipolar prostheses)
- Extracapsular fractures are generally treated with a dynamic hip screw or intramedullary device (for unstable ones)

Post-operative: multidisciplinary approach: physiotherapist, occupational therapist, social worker and family are involved

(Cx) Major blood supply to the head of the femur comes from the retinacular arteries, they are at particular risk with displaced intracapsular fractures and hence avascular necrosis

(Px) Mortality ~30 per cent at 1 year

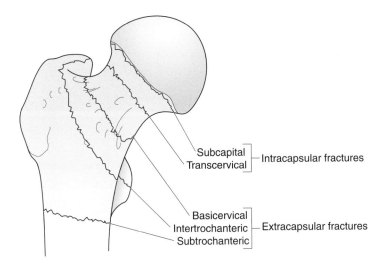

Figure 3.9 Common sites of fracture of the femoral neck

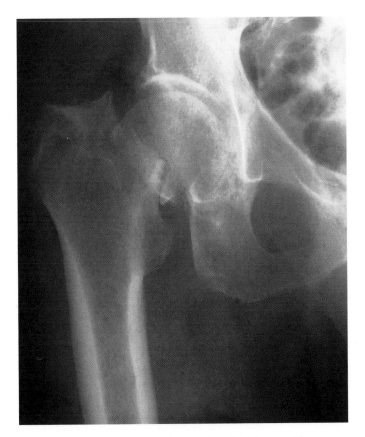

Figure 3.10 Intertrochanteric fractured neck of femur with displacement

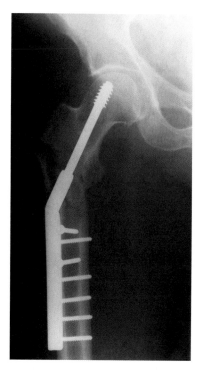

Figure 3.11 Post-operative insertion of a dynamic hip screw

ANTERIOR CRUCIATE LIGAMENT RUPTURE

A Acute knee swelling (haemarthrosis) with an associated rotational injury (e.g. rugby or skiing)

Si Positive anterior draw, Lachman's test ± pivot shift – difficult to assess acutely due to pain

Long-term: leg giving way, accelerated osteoarthritis (OA)

Ix *X-ray*: usually no fracture seen (rarely avulsion of the tibial spine)

MRI: investigation of choice to evaluate soft tissues

Arthroscopy: also assess associated meniscal injury

Rx See Table 3.2

Table 3.2 Treatment of anterior cruciate rupture

Non-operative	Operative (only if symptomatic or high-level)
Physiotherapy	Arthroscopy-assisted anterior cruciate ligament replacement with
Knee brace	autograft (patella tendon or hamstring tendon)
Walking aid	
Frequent spontaneous partial re-attachment	

TIBIAL PLATEAU FRACTURE

- Complicated fractures, caused by high-impact injuries
- Schatzker classification: Type I–VI
- Often need ORIF

TIBIAL FRACTURE

 P Often high-energy fractures, may involve extensive soft tissue damage

Rx Commonly treated with plaster, intramedullary nail or external fixation (Ilizarov frame)

Cx Watch out for compartment syndrome

Common peroneal nerve (CPN) involvement, if proximal fibula is fractured

CPN tests: sensation to first toe web space (superficial branch) and dorsiflexion of the great toe

ACHILLES TENDON RUPTURE

A Forced plantar flexion of the ankle

On systemic steroids

Sy Loud 'pop' and feeling of 'kicked in the back of the leg'

Tender, swelling ± gap in the Achilles tendon

Si Simmonds/Thompson test ('squeeze calf test') – absence of plantar flexion of the ankle

Ix Ultrasound scan/MRI

Rx *Non-operative*: plaster – full equinus

Operative: tendon repair and immobilization with plaster

ANKLE FRACTURES

A Common orthopaedic presentation to the emergency department

Ix Radiographs: mortice and lateral views of the ankle ± foot (if 5th metatarsal base fracture is suspected)

Box 3.2 DANIS–WEBER CLASSIFICATION OF ANKLE FRACTURES

There are three types depending on the level of fracture of the fibula
- *Type A*: below the syndesmosis
- *Type B*: at the level of the syndesmosis
- *Type C*: Above the syndesmosis

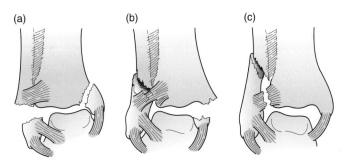

Figure 3.12 Danis–Weber classification of ankle fractures. There are three types depending on the level of the fracture of the fibula (a) Type A: below the syndesmosis (b) Type B: at the level of the syndesmosis (c) Type C: above the syndesmosis (reproduced with kind permission from Solomon L, Warwick DJ and Nayagam S, *Apley's Concise System of Orthopaedics and Fractures*, 3rd ed, Great Britain: Arnold, 2005)

Rx   *Danis–Weber A*: if undisplaced, walking cast is sufficient
Danis–Weber B: mostly need internal fixation, but sometimes treated with non-weight-bearing cast if undisplaced
Danis–Weber C: almost always unstable, needs internal fixation

ELECTIVE ORTHOPAEDICS

OSTEOARTHRITIS

(P) Degenerative disease of the joint characterized by breakdown of cartilage followed by new bone formation and capsular fibrosis

(Sy) Pain after exertion, stiffness, reduced range of movement and deformity
Secondary to fracture or congenital conditions (e.g. developmental dysplasia of the hip)

Box 3.3 RADIOGRAPHIC FEATURES OF OSTEOARTHRITIS

- **L**oss of joint space
- **O**steophytes
- **S**ubchondral cysts
- **S**clerosis

 Non-operative:
- – analgesia
- – lifestyle change
- – walking aid (if lower limb)
- – physiotherapy
- – occupational therapy
- – joint injection

- *Operative*:
  - – arthroscopy
  - – osteotomy (high tibial osteotomy for unicompartment OA of the knee)
  - – arthroplasty (total knee and hip replacement)
  - – arthrodesis (joint fusion)

LOWER LIMB ORTHOPAEDIC COMPLICATIONS

For clarity, the complications of total hip replacement are shown in Box 3.4.

Box 3.4 SPECIFIC COMPLICATIONS OF TOTAL HIP REPLACEMENT

- *Immediate*:
  - fat embolism
  - fracture of the femur or the acetabular floor
  - nerve damage (superior gluteal nerve, anterolateral approach; sciatic nerve, posterior approach)
  - haemorrhage
  - leg length difference
- *Early*:
  - infection (superficial and deep)
  - DVT/pulmonary embolism (PE)
  - leg length difference
  - dislocation
- *Late*:
  - aseptic loosening
  - periprosthetic fracture
  - bone stock loss
  - component fracture
  - ectopic ossification
  - late infection

BAKER'S CYST

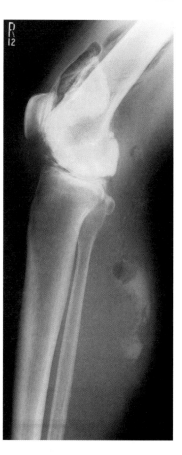

P   Posterior herniation of the knee joint capsule, secondary to OA

Si   Usually a painless swelling in the back of the knee, between the two heads of the gastrocnemius (beware of pulsatile swelling – popliteal aneurysm)
Ruptured Baker's cyst can be similar to DVT clinically

Ix   USS
Arthrogram (injection of contrast into knee to delineate capsule)

Rx   Aspiration occasionally for symptom relief
Treat as OA knee

Figure 3.13 Ruptured Baker's cyst: arthrography with injection of contrast and air into the knee joint; extravasation into the upper calf

LOWER BACK PAIN

 Common presentation to general practitioner (GP) and emergency department

 Sciatic pain: lower back pain radiating down one leg

Paraesthesiae to a dermatome

 Straight leg raise test – exacerbate pain or neurology

May present with other neurology

Wide differential diagnosis

- Night sweats and fever (consider TB)
- Sudden onset and collapse (rule out abdominal aortic aneurysm [AAA])
- Bilateral leg weakness and/or sphincter disturbance (bladder or bowel) – need urgent magnetic resonance imaging (MRI) to rule out cauda equina syndrome (see p. 162)

Box 3.5 CAUSES OF LOWER BACK PAIN

- *From the bone*:
  - mechanical back pain
  - spinal stenosis ('spinal claudication')
  - instability (spondylolisthesis)
  - infection (Potts' disease – TB of the spine)
  - tumour (primary, secondary)
  - multiple myeloma
  - referred pain from the hip
- *From the nerve*:
  - nerve root compression (radiculopathy)
- *From the intervertebral disc*:
  - prolapsed disc
  - infection (discitis)
  - degenerative disc
- *Connective tissue disease*:
  - ankylosing spondylitis
- *From the abdomen*:
  - abdominal aortic aneurysm
  - pancreatitis
  - renal stone

Ix According to suspected diagnosis

MRI is most useful for spinal pathology

Urgent computed tomography (CT) for suspected AAA

Rx *Conservative*:

- most mechanical back pain and disc prolapse can be treated conservatively
- physiotherapy, analgesia
- posture education

Operative treatment

- caudal epidural (equivocal evidence)
- discectomy
- spinal decompression
- spinal fusion
- intervertebral disc replacement

COMMON PAEDIATRIC CONDITIONS

DEVELOPMENTAL DYSPLASIA OF THE HIP (DDH)

P   Heterogeneous group, screening starts at birth, 6 weeks and 8 months

Sy   Difficulty walking, hip pain

Si   Asymmetrical skin crease, Barlow and Ortolani tests (attempted forced dislocation of hips)

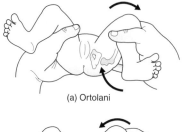

(a) Ortolani

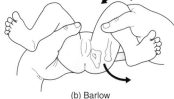

(b) Barlow   **Figure 3.14** (a) Ortolani test (b) Barlow test

Ix   USS of the hip (<5 months)

X-Ray – AP pelvis and frog lateral (>5 months)

Rx   Pavlik harness

Hip spica plaster cast

Open reduction

Complex pelvic and femoral osteotomies

PYOGENIC ARTHRITIS

A   Affects children under 2 years

P   Usually infection with *Staphylococcus*

S   Hip pain, septic

Ix   USS

Joint aspiration under anaesthesia – emergency

Rx   Joint washout

Antibiotics

PERTHES' DISEASE

P   Avascular necrosis of the femoral head of unknown aetiology

A   Affects children from 4–10 years

Sy   Hip pain, limp and referred knee pain

Ix   X-ray of the hips

Rx   Younger children require no treatment

Older children may need complex corrective operations including femoral osteotomies

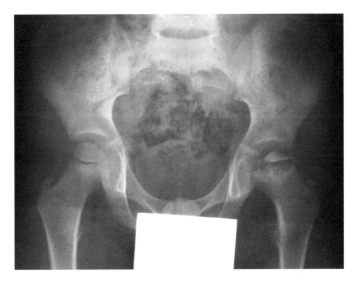

Figure 3.15 Perthes' disease: well established with flattening of the left femoral ossific nucleus and thickening of the femoral neck. A lead genital shield is in place

SLIPPED UPPER FEMORAL EPIPHYSIS

(A)   10–15 years, often obese males

(Sy)   Hip pain, limp and referred knee pain

(Ix)   X-ray: femoral head slipped over femoral neck (Klein's line or Trethowan's sign)

(Rx)   Cannulated screw

OSGOOD–SCHLATTER DISEASE

(S)   Active adolescent, pain on active extension, pain and prominence around the tibial tuberosity

(Ix)   X-ray: partial fragmentation of the tibial apophysis

(Rx)   Rest

    Resolution in 1–2 years

BONE TUMOURS

See Table 3.3

Table 3.3 Bone tumours

Origin	Benign	Malignant
Primary		
Cartilage	Chondroma	Chondrosarcoma
Bone	Osteoid osteoma	Osteosarcoma
Fibrous tissue	Fibroma	Fibrosarcoma
	Myxoid fibroma	
Vascular	Haemangioma	Angiosarcoma
Secondary		
Breast		
Bronchus		
Prostate		
Kidney		
Thyroid		

Ear, nose and throat

Alex Charkin

EARS

OTITIS EXTERNA

- **(P)** Inflammation of the skin of the external auditory meatus (ear canal)
- **(A)** May be caused by bacteria (commonly *Staphylococcus* or *Pseudomonas*) or fungi
- **(Sy)** Irritation, pain, discharge and deafness (canal becomes blocked with debris)
- **(Si)** Tenderness upon moving the ear, moist debris, which when removed reveals an erythematous canal
- **(Rx)** Microsuction and topical antibiotic and steroid drops. If the canal is very oedematous, insert wick to splint open canal and allow drops into ear

ACUTE OTITIS MEDIA

- **(P)** Acute inflammation of the middle ear cavity, highest incidence in children (3–7 years old)
- **(A)** May be primary infection or secondary following an upper respiratory tract infection (common)
  Causative organisms *Streptococcus pneumoniae*, *Haemophilus influenza* and *Moraxella catarrhalis*
- **(Sy)** Otalgia (sudden relief if tympanic membrane perforates with release of pus), decreased hearing in affected ear
- **(Si)** Fever, bulging, red tympanic membrane, sometimes fluid level visible behind membrane
- **(Ix)** Full blood count (FBC)
- **(Rx)** Antibiotics and analgesia
- **(Cx)** Mastoiditis, meningitis, intracranial abscesses, lateral sinus thrombosis

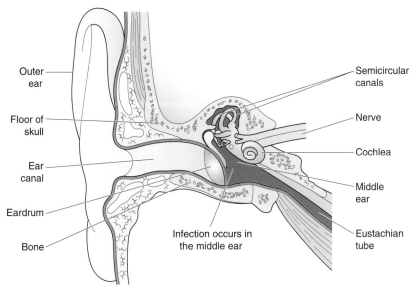

Figure 4.1 Otitis media (diagram source copyright EMIS and PiP as distributed on http://www.patient.co.uk)

MASTOIDITIS

 Follows acute otitis media

 Tenderness ± erythema overlying mastoid, displacement of the ear forward and a red or bulging tympanic membrane (NB if normal then the patient does not have mastoiditis)

 Antibiotics and if evidence of an abscess or no response with antibiotics, then surgery, i.e. mastoidectomy

OTITIS MEDIA WITH EFFUSION ('GLUE EAR')

 Characterized by fluid in the middle ear resulting in conductive deafness
Underlying cause: Eustachian tube dysfunction, e.g. secondary to large adenoids. Middle ear pressure falls, inflammation results and copious, tenacious mucus forms

 Vast majority of cases occur in children, most present between 3 and 6 years old and are worse during the winter

 Deafness. Less commonly speech and language delay, otalgia and recurrent infections

 Dull, retracted tympanic membrane

 Audiogram and tympanogram (compliance falls with middle ear fluid). In adults the post-nasal space should be visualized to exclude a tumour, especially if unilateral

 Grommet insertion (ventilation tubes) if spontaneous resolution does not occur. Often combined with adenoidectomy

---

INFORMATION BOX: TYMPANOGRAM

A tympanogram is a specialist investigation used to look at the movement of the tympanic membrane when a blast of air hits it. A graph is produced of the movement – this can show decreased compliance in diseases such as glue ear where fluid prevents proper movement of the membrane (see Fig. 4.2)

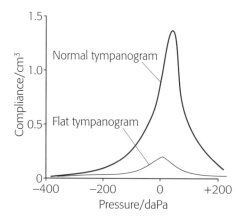

Figure 4.2 Normal and flat tympanogram, demonstrating reduced tympanic membrane compliance in otitis media with effusion

CHOLESTEATOMA

P Stratified squamous epithelial cells within the middle ear cleft, independently growing and causing local destruction often with superadded infection

A May be congenital or acquired

Sy Foul-smelling discharge

Si Otoscopy reveals pearly white mass

Ix Audiogram and computed tomography (CT) scan

Rx Surgical excision

Cx Facial nerve (VII) palsy, meningitis and cerebral abscess formation

Px Good resolution with correct operation

MÉNIÈRE'S DISEASE

P Also known as endolymphatic hydrops, where there is ↑ pressure in the endolymph of the inner ear

A ♀ = ♂; occurs in early to late adulthood

Sy Triad of episodic vertigo, tinnitus and deafness. Often associated with a sensation of fullness in the ear

Si Vomiting, nystagmus

Ix Audiogram may show low-frequency hearing loss after repeated attacks

Rx *Medical*: labyrinthine vasodilator e.g. betahistine, vestibular sedatives e.g. prochlorperazine and diuretics
Surgery: Grommet insertion (possible placebo effect), decompression and vestibular nerve section

PINNA HAEMATOMA

P Traumatic collection of blood between the cartilage and the perichondrium, from which it takes its blood supply

A Prompt treatment is needed to prevent permanent deformity ('cauliflower ear' – common in boxers)

S Swollen, painful ear with fluctuant collection

Aseptic evacuation of the haematoma with subsequent compression to prevent recollection

OTALGIA

If the ears look normal consider referred pain from the following:

- *teeth* (auriculo-temporal branch of the trigeminal nerve)
- *herpes zoster* i.e. Ramsay–Hunt Syndrome (sensory branch of facial nerve), pain
- *throat* e.g. tonsillitis or base of tongue (tympanic branch of glossopharyngeal)
- *larynx* e.g. carcinoma (auricular branch of the vagus)
- *neck and cervical discs* (great auricular nerve (C2–3) and lesser occipital nerve [C2])

NOSE

EPISTAXIS

(P) Haemorrhage from the nose

Most recurrent epistaxis is from the anterior part of the septum (Little's area)

(A) Anterior bleeding is more common in the young, posterior bleeding more often seen in the elderly

---

Box 4.1 CAUSES OF EPISTAXIS

- *Local*:
  - idiopathic
  - trauma
  - tumours
- *Systemic*:
  - anticoagulants
  - bleeding disorders
  - hypertension
  - Osler–Weber–Rendu disease/hereditary haemorrhagic telangiectasia (rare)

(S) Nose bleed (occasionally shock or haematemesis)

(Ix) Direct inspection of nose ± clotting screen

(Rx) Cautery (with silver nitrate), nasal packing. For refractory bleeding surgery with artery ligation or radiological embolization may be required

(Cx) Hypotension, shock

SINUSITIS

(P) Inflammation and infection of the sinuses, maybe acute or chronic.

Any one or all of the four pairs may be affected

(A) Usually secondary to viral upper respiratory tract infection (URTI). Maxillary sinusitis may be dental in origin e.g. dental root abscess

(Sy) Pain over sinuses, nasal obstruction, preceding URTI

(Si) Fever, tenderness over sinuses, mucopus in middle meatus; NB swelling over the cheek is rare in maxillary sinusitis, swelling over the frontal sinus may be secondary to frontal osteomyelitis

(Ix) CT scan (plain radiograph may demonstrate opaque sinuses)

(Rx) Antibiotics, nasal vasoconstrictors. In chronic disease, operative enlargement of the sinus drainage opening

(Cx) Orbital cellulitis or abscess, meningitis, intracranial abscess, osteomyelitis of the frontal bone ('Potts puffy tumour')

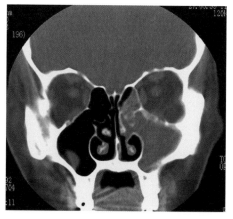

Figure 4.3 Coronal CT with polypoidal mucosal thickening in the right maxillary antrum and complete opacification on the left

RHINITIS

(P) Inflammatory hypersensitivity of the nasal mucosa

(A) Either allergic or non-allergic

(Sy) Rhinorrhoea, nasal obstruction, sneezing

(Si) Copious mucous, oedematous nasal mucosa, transverse nasal skin crease (in children who continuously rub their nose)

(Ix) Skin prick testing, radioallergosorbent test (RAST) (allergy testing)

(Rx) Avoid allergen, antihistamines (cetirizine/chlorphenamine), topical steroid spray, vasoconstrictor nasal drops (short term only)

NASAL POLYPS

(P) Abnormal lesions from the nasal mucosa or paranasal sinuses

(A) Usually ♂ and over 40 years old

If present in children a diagnosis of cystic fibrosis must be considered

(Sy) Asymptomatic, nasal obstruction, rhinorrhoea, post-nasal drip, hyposmia

(Si) Pale fleshy polyps seen usually arising from the middle meatus (may need nasendoscopy). If large they may protrude out of the nose

(Rx) *Medical*: topical ± oral steroids

Surgery: endoscopic sinus surgery and polypectomy

THROAT

TONSILLITIS

(P) Inflammation of the tonsils (pharyngeal), part of Waldeyer's lymphoid tissue ring

(A) Causative organisms:
- *bacterial*: β-haemolytic *Streptococcus*, *S. pneumoniae*, *H. influenzae*
- *viral*: influenza, parainfluenza, adenovirus

(Sy) Malaise and sore throat with odynophagia (pain on swallowing) with or without otalgia (ear ache)

(Si) Fever, inflamed and enlarged tonsils with exudate, cervical lymphadenopathy
Differential diagnosis: glandular fever, caused by Epstein–Barr virus has similar presentation

(Ix) Full blood count ± Monospot test (for glandular fever)

(Rx) Analgesia, penicillin (treats bacterial infection and prevents superadded infection with viral tonsillitis), may require intravenous (i.v.) fluids if unable to swallow
Careful with amoxicillin – if patient has glandular fever the drug causes a widespread maculopapular rash

(Cx) See Box 4.2

Box 4.2 COMPLICATIONS OF TONSILLITIS

- *General*:
  - septicaemia
  - rheumatic fever
  - post-streptococcal acute glomerulonephritis
- *Local*:
  - respiratory obstruction
  - abscess formation

(Px) Consider tonsillectomy for recurrent attacks over several years

QUINSY (PERITONSILLAR ABSCESS)

(P) Pus around the fibrous capsule of the tonsil, in the soft tissues
Sequela of tonsillitis

(Sy) Preceding sore throat, increasing unilateral pain with otalgia, difficulty swallowing

(Si) 'Hot potato speech' (soft palate splinting), spitting out saliva, trismus ('lock-jaw') medialization of a tonsil, deviation of uvula away and soft palate swelling

(Rx) Aspiration ± incision, i.v. antibiotics

(Px) Tonsillectomy as above or if recurrent quinsy

EPIGLOTTITIS/SUPRAGLOTTITIS

(P) Bacterial infection of the supraglottis (area above the vocal cords), which may predominantly affect the epiglottis

(A) Epiglottitis usually affects children (3–4 years old) and supraglottitis usually adults
Usually *Haemophilus influenzae*, sometimes *Streptococcus*

(Sy) Odynophagia (painful swallowing), dysphagia

Si Fever, hoarse voice, drooling, stridor or *in extremis* with airway compromise

Ix In adults visualization of the larynx with either a mirror or nasendoscope

Rx Assess and secure airway as required, i.e. intubate or tracheostomy

NB if suspected in children **do not attempt to examine** (may precipitate airway obstruction), call for senior anaesthetist, i.v. antibiotics (third generation cephalosporin) and dexamethasone

STRIDOR

P High-pitched sound made by turbulent flow through a partially obstructed airway

It is a sign, not a diagnosis

A *Congenital*: laryngomalacia, vocal cord palsy, tracheomalacia

Acquired: epiglottitis/supraglottitis, croup, foreign body, vocal cord palsy, trauma, allergy

Si Harsh, noisy breathing; cyanosis; collapse

Ix Lateral soft tissue neck, fibre optic nasendoscopy

Rx Oxygen, nebulized adrenaline, dexamethasone

Conservative, i.e. observe, or secure airway e.g. intubate/tracheostomy and treat cause

CHAPTER 5

Urology

Simon Bott and Ben Eddy

THE ACUTE SCROTUM

TESTICULAR TORSION

(P) *Intravaginal*: rotation within tunica vaginalis, usually peripubertal
Extravaginal: rotation on the spermatic cord, usually neonates

(Sy) Acute onset pain in the testis ± iliac fossa, nausea and vomiting, often previous similar episodes with spontaneous resolution.

(Si) Tender swollen testis, overlying scrotal skin may be red
Cremasteric reflex may be absent on affected side

(Ix) Doppler ultrasound scan may show ↓ arterial flow, but must not delay definitive treatment

(Rx) Urgent scrotal exploration, untwist testis
Both testes fixed; if the testis is infarcted orchidectomy and fixation of contralateral testis
Differential diagnosis: orchitis, torsion of hydatid of Morgagni, strangulated inguinal hernia, testis tumour

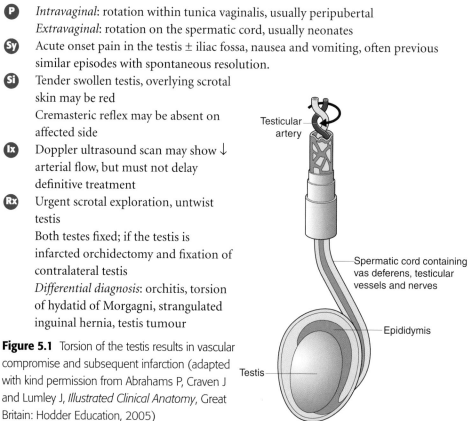

Figure 5.1 Torsion of the testis results in vascular compromise and subsequent infarction (adapted with kind permission from Abrahams P, Craven J and Lumley J, *Illustrated Clinical Anatomy*, Great Britain: Hodder Education, 2005)

Testicular artery

Spermatic cord containing vas deferens, testicular vessels and nerves

Epididymis

Testis

EPIDIDYMO-ORCHITIS

(A) Typically *Chlamydia* in sexually active young men and *E. coli* in older men,
May be viral orchitis – mumps, Coxsackie, infective mononucleosis, or bacterial
epididymo-orchitis – *Gonococcus*, TB

(Sy) Unilateral or bilateral testis pain, swelling, fever, frequency, dysuria

(Si) Tender swollen testis, overlying scrotal skin is red

(Ix) Doppler ultrasound scan (USS) may show ↑ arterial flow

(Rx) Once torsion has been excluded treatment is with antibiotics (ofloxacin)

TORSION OF THE HYDATID OF MORGAGNI

(P) Embryological remnant, which can twist and infarct

(A) Usually in pre-pubescent boys

(Sy) Similar to testicular torsion

(Si) May see 'blue-dot' sign through scrotal skin, non-tender testis

(Rx) Usually requires scrotal exploration to exclude torsion

THE PROSTATE

BENIGN PROSTATIC HYPERPLASIA (BPH)

(A) Affects men over 50 years, incidence ↑ with age

(S) *Voiding*: hesitancy, poor stream, incomplete bladder emptying, pis-en-deux (large second voiding of urine immediately after finishing normal urination)

Storage: frequency, nocturia, urgency

Abdominal examination is usually unremarkable, may palpate an enlarged bladder and *per rectum* (PR) examination will reveal an enlarged prostate

(Ix) Full blood count (FBC) – anaemia in renal failure, urea and electrolytes (U&E), mid-stream urine (MSU)

Urinary flow rate and post-void residual urine volume

Consider prostate-specific antigen PSA (? carcinoma), urodynamic investigation

(Rx) See Box 5.1

Box 5.1 TREATMENT OPTIONS IN BENIGN PROSTATIC HYPERPLASIA

- *Conservative*:
  - avoid caffeinated and sugary drinks and evening fluids
- *Medical*:
  - α-blocker e.g. tamsulosin or alfuzosin
  - 5α-reductase inhibitor e.g. finasteride or dutasteride (prevents peripheral activation of testosterone in prostate)
- *Surgery*:
  - trans-urethral resection of the prostate (TURP), laser vaporization or enucleation

---

(Cx) Acute urinary retention, overflow incontinence, acute renal failure, bladder stones, recurrent UTI and haematuria

Acute retention requires urgent catheterization; record residual urine and whether creatinine is elevated, watch for a diuresis (urine output >200 mL/h), replace with normal saline as necessary

PROSTATE CANCER

(A) 40 per cent of males born in the Western world will develop prostate cancer

10 per cent will be diagnosed with it

3 per cent will die from the disease

Incidence ↓ in Asia, but approaches Western levels in Asian immigrants living in the US. ↑ incidence in African–American men

Risk factors include aging and positive family history (one first-degree relative 2× risk, two first-degree relatives 5× risk)

(Sy) Storage and voiding symptoms (see BPH), haematuria/spermia,

(Si) Hard nodular prostate on rectal exam

Occasional incidental diagnosis after TURP

Can also present with advanced disease – acute renal failure from ureteric obstruction, bone pain, pathological fracture, spinal cord compression, malaise, weight loss

PSA (can monitor course of disease), FBC, U&E, Ca^{2+}, liver function tests (LFT)
Transrectal ultrasound-guided prostatic biopsy – provides Gleason grading
Magnetic resonance imaging (MRI) to assess if cancer is prostate confined or there is
lymph node involvement
Nuclear medicine bone scan (? metastases)

INFORMATION BOX: TNM (TUMOUR, NODE, METASTASIS) (2000) STAGING OF PROSTATE CANCER

- *T1*: impalpable and not visible on imaging
- *T2*: tumour confined within the prostate
- *T3*: tumour extends outside the prostate capsule
- *T4*: tumour invades adjacent structures (bladder, pelvic wall, levator ani)

Box 5.2 TREATMENT OPTIONS IN PROSTATE CANCER

- *Localized disease* (prostate confined):
  - active surveillance: monitor PSA and treat if PSA rises or cancer upgraded on repeat biopsy
  - radiotherapy: external beam or brachytherapy (^{125}Iodine seed implantation)
  - surgery: laparoscopic or open radical prostatectomy
- *Advanced disease*:
  - medical: hormonal manipulation with gonadotrophin-releasing hormone (GnRH) agonist (goserelin, leuprorelin, triptorelin) or testosterone antagonist (flutamide, bicalutamide)
  - radiotherapy: treat painful bone metastases

PROSTATITIS

 Complex of symptoms and aetiologies, 50 per cent of men will experience
symptoms during lifetime.
- *category 1*: acute infection of the prostate (*E. coli, Pseudomonas, Klebsiella*)
- *category 2*: chronic infection of the prostate (*E. coli, Pseudomonas, Klebsiella*)
- *category 3*: chronic pelvic pain syndrome (without infection but with or without inflammation)
- *category 4*: asymptomatic inflammatory prostatitis (incidental finding) after TURP/prostate biopsy

 Pelvic, urethral, perineal or rectal pain, frequency, urgency. If category 1 there may
be life-threatening septicaemia and urinary retention

PR may reveal exquisitely tender, boggy prostate

Pyuria on MSU. Diagnosis confirmed by prostatic massage and microscopy and
culture of prostatic secretions

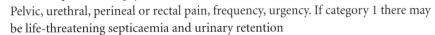 3–4 weeks of fluoroquinolone (ciprofloxacin/ofloxacin) treatment, or TURP if
abscess. Retention should be treated with suprapubic catheterization
Category 3: notoriously difficult to treat – may get response with α-blocker, non-
steroidal anti-inflammatory drugs (NSAIDs), long-term antibiotics, diazepam,
prostatic massage, warm baths, avoiding caffeine, alcohol and spicy food,
reassurance that it is not life-threatening
Category 4: needs no treatment

HAEMATURIA

BLADDER CANCER

(A) 12 000 new cases per annum in UK, ♂:♀ 3:1

Risk factors include smoking and exposure to aromatic amines (industries include clothing dyes, printing, petrochemical and aluminium smelting)

Mean age at diagnosis is 65 years

(P) Latency period after exposure can be up to 20 years

90 per cent are transitional cell carcinoma (TCC)

80 per cent present with superficial disease, 20 per cent have invasive disease

Small proportion are squamous cell carcinoma (risk factors include schistosomiasis, chronic infection, long term catheterization)

(Sy) Haematuria most common presenting symptom

Macroscopic haematuria has 25 per cent risk of TCC

Microscopic haematuria has 5 per cent risk of TCC

Can also present with recurrent UTIs and storage symptoms (frequency, urgency)

(Ix) *Endoscopy*: flexible cystoscopy is gold standard

Imaging: USS and intravenous urogram (IVU) to look for upper tract disease

Computed tomography (CT) useful for extravesical spread

Pathology: Urine cytology useful in high-grade disease

INFORMATION BOX: TNM STAGING OF BLADDER CANCER

Superficial disease
- *Ta*: non-invasive papillary
- *Tis*: carcinoma *in situ*
- *T1*: tumour invades lamina propria

Invasive disease
- *T2*: tumour invades muscle
- *T3*: tumour extends outside bladder
- *T4*: tumour invades adjacent organs

(Rx) *Superficial disease*:
- endoscopic resection, examination under anaesthesia (EUA) and intravesical chemotherapy to reduce recurrence
- patients need regular surveillance cystoscopies

Invasive disease:
- radical cystectomy (50 per cent 5-year survival) or radical radiotherapy (40 per cent 5-year survival)
- prognosis is related to stage of initial disease

(Px) Overall mortality of 23 per cent for all stages and grades of disease

URINARY STONE DISEASE (UROLITHIASIS)

(A) Increasing incidence over last 50 years

Prevalence of 2 per cent, lifetime risk of 1 in 8 ♂:♀ 3:1

Most common in 4th and 5th decade, 10 per cent bilateral

High incidence in USA, UK and Scandinavia, low incidence in Africa and South America

---

Box 5.3 CAUSES OF RENAL STONES

- Idiopathic
- Infection
- Obstruction
- Prolonged immobilization
- Hot climate
- Hyperparathyroidism
- Oral calcium supplements
- Congenital abnormalities (i.e. horseshoe kidney and duplex systems)
- Genetic (positive family history in 25 per cent)
- Sedentary occupation

(P) *Stone type*:
- 90 per cent are calcium based therefore are radio-opaque
- urate stones (5 per cent) are radiolucent, so will not show up on abdominal X-ray

(Sy) Severe loin pain (10/10 intensity). Pain radiating to the iliac fossa, testis, penile tip or labia suggests a mid or distal ureteric stone

Differential diagnosis: appendicitis, abdominal aortic aneurysm (AAA), biliary colic, diverticulitis, torted ovarian cyst or torted testis

(Ix) *Urinalysis*: 97 per cent will have microscopic haematuria, if absent then a stone is unlikely

Bloods : FBC, U&E, Ca^{2+}, PO_4^{3-}, urate

Imaging:
- IVU is the gold standard, look for enhanced nephrogram, delayed excretion, hydronephrosis, hydroureter and standing column
- common sites of obstruction include the pelvic–ureteric junction (PUJ), pelvic brim and vesico–ureteric junction (VUJ)
- non-contrast CT urogram, very sensitive for stone disease and useful alternative

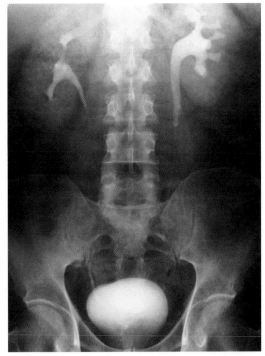

Figure 5.2 IVU showing obstruction of the left kidney from a ureteric calculus

Analgesia, NSAIDs/opiates

Small stones <6 mm will usually pass spontaneously (80 per cent),

Larger stones or complete obstruction – ureteric stent

Emergency percutaneous nephrostomy if septic and obstructed

Ureteric stones can be treated with ureteroscopy and stone fragmentation (laser)

Small (<2 cm) renal stones managed with extracorporeal shockwave lithotripsy (ESWL)

Large (>2 cm) renal stones managed by percutaneous nephrolithotomy

 50 per cent will recur within 10 years

THE KIDNEY

RENAL TUMOURS

A   3 per cent of all adult cancers worldwide

♂:♀ 2:1

Average age at diagnosis 70 years

High incidence in the West, low incidence in Asian countries, cause unknown

Risk factors include smoking, obesity and chronic renal disease needing dialysis

P   Majority are adenocarcinomas, known as renal cell carcinoma (RCC)

Familial variant of RCC known as von Hippel–Lindau disease

S   Haematuria seen in 40 per cent

Classic triad of loin pain, haematuria, palpable mass rarely occurs (<10 per cent), and usually indicates advanced disease

Anaemia, polycythaemia, hypercalcaemia, hypertension, malaise, fever or unexplained weight loss

50 per cent detected incidentally as a result of increased use of imaging techniques

Cx   Local disease can spread to renal vein, inferior vena cava (IVC) or surrounding structures (e.g. adrenal)

Metastatic disease commonly to bones, lung (cannon ball lesions) and lymph nodes

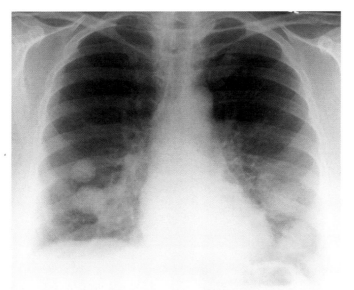

Figure 5.3 Multiple lung metastases secondary to renal carcinoma

Ix   USS more sensitive than IVU for renal lesions

CT is the gold standard for imaging and staging local and metastatic disease

Bone scan if symptomatic or raised alkaline phosphatase (ALP)

INFORMATION BOX: TNM STAGING OF RENAL TUMOURS

- *T1*: tumour <7 cm confined to the kidney
- *T2*: tumour >7 cm confined to the kidney
- *T3*: extends beyond the kidney, i.e. renal vein, IVC or adrenal gland
- *T4*: extends beyond Gerota's fascia (connective tissue capsule of the kidney)

(Rx) Laparoscopic or open radical nephrectomy is the treatment of choice
Surgery for metastatic disease in selected cases
Tumours are chemo- and radio-insensitive so these therapies have limited role,
immunotherapy (interferon/interleukins) for selected metastatic cases

(Px) 90 per cent 5-year survival for T1 disease
0–13 per cent 5-year survival for metastatic disease

COMMON PRESENTATIONS

HAEMATURIA

A Very common problem, may be a sign of serious underlying disease

10 per cent of urology referrals

Overall prevalence 5 per cent, up to 20 per cent in those aged over 60 years

P See Fig. 5.4

S Microscopic or macroscopic haematuria

Painful haematuria suggests infection

Pain at start of stream suggests prostatic or urethral origin

Loin pain suggests renal origin

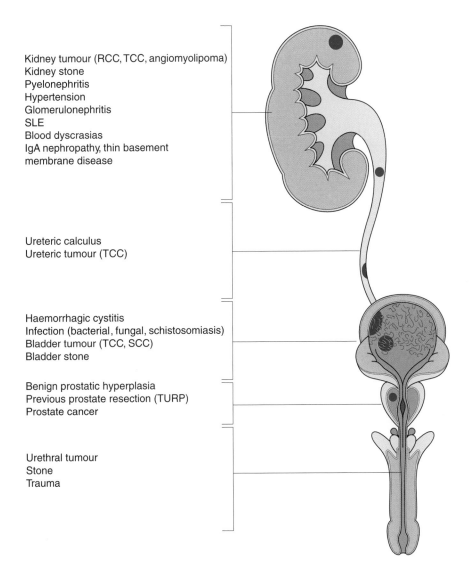

Kidney tumour (RCC, TCC, angiomyolipoma)
Kidney stone
Pyelonephritis
Hypertension
Glomerulonephritis
SLE
Blood dyscrasias
IgA nephropathy, thin basement
membrane disease

Ureteric calculus
Ureteric tumour (TCC)

Haemorrhagic cystitis
Infection (bacterial, fungal, schistosomiasis)
Bladder tumour (TCC, SCC)
Bladder stone

Benign prostatic hyperplasia
Previous prostate resection (TURP)
Prostate cancer

Urethral tumour
Stone
Trauma

Figure 5.4 Causes of haematuria

Ⓘx *Microscopic* (confirmed on two freshly voided urines without infection):
– if aged over 40 years will need MSU/urine cytology/U&E/PSA (prostate-specific antigen)/IVU (or kidneys, ureters and bladder (KUB) X-ray and USS) and flexible cystoscopy
– investigate if under 40 years if there are risk factors in history i.e. smoking
– consider renal referral if there is evidence of casts, dysmorphic cells, proteinuria, hypertension or an elevated creatinine

Macroscopic (visible to the naked eye):
– all patients should be investigated
– MSU/urine cytology/U&E/PSA/IVU/renal USS and flexible cystoscopy
– if all normal probably prostatic in origin, however if persistent consider CT/magnetic resonance imaging (MRI) or renal angiogram as vascular malformations are rare causes
– novel markers for bladder cancer like NMP-22 appear promising but are not in clinical use yet
– patients may need admission for bladder washouts/transfusion or general anaesthetic cystoscopy and washout in severe cases

URINARY TRACT INFECTION

Ⓐ Very common health problem
Usually as a result of bacterial ascent along urethra
More common in women, due to shorter urethra, moist environment and proximity to anus

---

Box 5.4 PREDISPOSING FACTORS TO URINARY TRACT INFECTION

- Stones
- Foreign bodies (e.g. catheters)
- Congenital abnormalities (e.g. duplex system, horseshoe kidney, PUJ obstruction)
- Bladder outflow obstruction from BPH or strictures
- Other diseases including TCC or fistulae from adjacent organs

---

Ⓟ Common organisms include *E. coli*, *Proteus* spp, *Pseudomonas* spp, *Klebsiella* and *Enterococcus*

Ⓢ Can be asymptomatic
Cystitis: frequency, urgency, dysuria and suprapubic pain, fever is unusual
Pyelonephritis: loin pain, nausea, fever (temp >38°C), rigors and a leucocytosis

Ⓘx Investigate all men, recurrent infections, children and infections in pregnancy
Urinalysis: protein, leucocytes and nitrites indicate infection
MSU:
– microscopy and culture should be used to confirm infection prior to starting antibiotics
– >10^3 colony-forming units (CFUs) in uncomplicated and >10^5 CFUs in complicated UTI is diagnostic
Imaging:
– KUB X-ray to rule out stone disease
– renal USS to identify reflux and renal scarring

- consider DMSA (nuclear medicine scan) if scarring seen

Endoscopy: cystoscopy rarely useful in young patients unless there are other risk factors e.g. haematuria

 Conservative measures first, increase fluid intake, hygiene advice, double voiding, emptying bladder after intercourse, cranberry juice

Asymptomatic UTI: needs no treatment (except in pregnancy)

Uncomplicated UTI: 3-day course of antibiotics usually adequate

Recurrent infections: consider prophylactic antibiotics, rotated 3 monthly

Pyelonephritis: needs 2 week course (exclude other causes first)

Antibiotics:
- first-line trimethoprim or amoxicillin (high resistance rates in hospitals)
- second-line consider a quinolone (ciprofloxacin) or cephalosporin (cefalexin) – obtain sensitivities before starting treatment if possible

IMPOTENCE

 Common problem, increasing incidence with age

Wide variety of causes (see Box 5.5)

Box 5.5 CAUSES OF IMPOTENCE

- *Neurological*: autonomic neuropathy (usually secondary to diabetes), multiple sclerosis and spinal injuries
- *Vascular*: pelvic/aorto-iliac disease
- *Iatrogenic*: commonly α- and β-blockers, psychotropic agents
- *Alcohol abuse*
- *Psychological*: depression
- *Endocrine*: hyperprolactinaemia, hypo/hyperthyroidism, Cushing's syndrome, androgen deficiency

---

 Loss of libido is a sign of androgen deficiency and hyperprolactinaemia

Spontaneous morning erections with impotence are suggestive of psychogenic disease

 Treat underlying disease if possible

Phosphodiesterase inhibitors (sildenafil) improve penile blood flow via nitric oxide

Testosterone treatment if there is proven hypogonadism

CHAPTER 6

Ophthalmology

Jagdeep Singh Gandhi

In finals in ophthalmology examiners are fond of only a few subjects such as diabetic and hypertensive retinopathy, the appearances of the optic disc, and III, IV and VI nerve palsies.

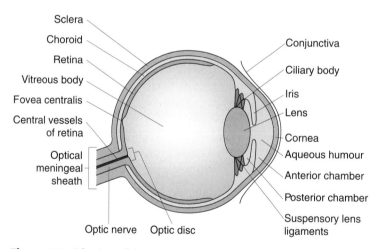

Sclera
Choroid
Retina
Vitreous body
Fovea centralis
Central vessels of retina
Optical meningeal sheath
Optic nerve   Optic disc

Conjunctiva
Ciliary body
Iris
Lens
Cornea
Aqueous humour
Anterior chamber
Posterior chamber
Suspensory lens ligaments

Figure 6.1 Side view of the eye (adapted with kind permission from Abrahams P, Craven J and Lumley J, *Illustrated Clinical Anatomy*, Great Britain: Hodder Education, 2005)

THE RED EYE

CONJUNCTIVITIS

 Inflammation of the conjunctiva

A *Infections*:
- viral (most cases e.g. adenovirus, herpes simplex),
- bacterial (e.g. *Staphylococcus*, *Streptococcus*), *Chlamydia* (in young sexually active patients)

Allergic: commonly seasonal

Toxins: chemical splash, chlorine

Radiation: direct irritation of conjunctival tissue

Trauma: blinking of very dry eyes

Sy Uncomfortable (typically **not** painful) eye, vision typically normal

Si Redness, sticky discharge, swollen eyelids: follicles (typically in infection) or papillae (typically in allergy), seen as lumps when lid is everted

Ix Usually a self-limiting condition. Conjunctival swabs and viral cultures if persistent, or very severe

Rx Chloramphenicol gives broad-spectrum, bacteriostatic cover. Frequently, ocular lubricants ('artificial tears') alone are adequate and provide symptomatic relief

CORNEAL ULCER

A *Infections*: viral (herpes simplex: 'dendritic' ulcer), bacterial (*Staphylococcus*, *Streptococcus*), rarely fungal

Cold sores (herpes simplex virus [HSV]), contact lens wear, lid margin disease (blepharitis)

Sy Pain, photophobia, blurred vision, sensation of foreign body

Si Red eye, corneal opacity, corneal stain with fluorescein, hypopyon (sediment of white cells in the anterior chamber)

Ix If the ulcer is severe or persistent then scrape-samples are taken from the cornea for microscopy, culture and sensitivities (MC&S) analysis

Rx *Herpes simplex infections*: aciclovir ointment

Bacterial keratitis: topical antibiotics

Topical steroids added only when microbiology is known or there is clinical improvement

IRITIS

 Inflammation of the iris is a common ophthalmic presentation

 Most cases are idiopathic (>95 per cent)

Remainder are associated with systemic conditions (human leucocyte antigen [HLA]-B27, ankylosing spondylitis, sarcoid, TB, etc.), or an intrinsic eye problem (e.g. corneal ulcer, retinal detachment, etc.)

Sy Pain, photophobia, blurred vision

Si Redness often around the cornea, cells in the anterior chamber, pupil stuck to lens in parts, clumps of cells stuck to inner surface of cornea, ↑ or ↓ intraocular pressure

Ix Screening tests for systemic conditions if iritis is recurrent, severe or bilateral

 Topical steroid, cycloplegic/mydriatic (dilating) drops (e.g. cyclopentolate, atropine)

EPISCLERITIS

(P) Usually a self-limiting inflammation of the connective tissue layer overlying the sclera

(A) Most cases idiopathic
Some associated with dry eyes, contact lens wear, rarely rheumatological disease

(Sy) Sore, irritable eye, foreign body sensation

(Si) Localized redness

(Rx) Topical steroid/lubricants given if symptomatic

SCLERITIS

(P) Severe inflammation of the sclera that can potentially result in necrosis and perforation in some cases

(A) Frequently associated with rheumatological disease and vasculitides

(Sy) Deep, boring, severe pain

(Si) Exquisite tenderness

(Ix) Rheumatological and vasculitic screen (e.g. rheumatoid factor [RhF], inflammatory markers, full blood count (FBC), antineutrophil cytoplasmic antibodies [ANCA])

(Rx) Intensive topical/local steroid, systemic non-steroidal anti-inflammatory drugs (NSAIDs) and steroids

ACUTE ANGLE-CLOSURE GLAUCOMA

(A) Important cause of a painful red eye in the older (50+ years) patient

(P) Affected eyes have an anatomical predisposition: shallow anterior chamber

(Sy) Intermittent eye pain, headache, haloes (corneal oedema), blurred vision, severe pain, nausea and vomiting (during acute angle-closure)

(Si) Red eye, mid-dilated oval pupil, shallow anterior chamber, corneal oedema, other eye also has shallow anterior chamber

(Ix) Gonioscopy (special lens examination) shows an occluded iridocorneal angle in the affected eye and an at-risk configuration in the other eye's angle

(Rx) *Medical*: aimed at lower intraocular pressure with systemic and topical antiglaucoma drugs, e.g. mannitol, pilocarpine
Surgical: peripheral laser iridotomy done to prevent further attack of angle-closure

DIABETIC RETINOPATHY

(A) Long-standing diabetes, related to poor glycaemic control

(P) Basic problem is damage to the blood–retina barrier
This damage causes occlusion or leakage in the retinal circulation
Diabetic retinopathy consists of a spectrum of lesions

Box 6.1 CLASSIFICATION OF DIABETIC RETINOPATHY

Background retinopathy:
- **H**aemorrhage:
  - leakage of blood into the retina
  - dot, blot, flame-shaped haemorrhages
- **O**edema:
  - leakage of fluid (transudate)
  - diabetic macular oedema can occur even in background disease
- **M**icroaneurysms:
  - outpouchings of venous end of capillaries
  - earliest sign of retinopathy, found in the central macula
- **E**xudates:
  - leakage of lipid
  - yellowish deposits, usually in the macula

Pre-proliferative retinopathy
- *Cotton wool spot:*
  - with blockage of fine retinal capillaries (axoplasmic) flow is slowed, producing a feathery whitish area called a 'cotton wool spot' – this represents a focal infarct
- *Vein abnormalities:*
  - characterize an ischaemic retina
  - venous looping, beading and engorgement can be seen

Proliferative retinopathy
- New vessel growth from the retina
- New vessel growth from the optic disc
- New vessel growth from the iris (rubeosis)

Advanced retinopathy
- Scar tissue is laid down inside the eye
- Tractional retinal detachment (scar tissue associated with neovascular processes pulls on the retina)
- Retinal gliosis (scarring)
- Vitreous haemorrhage

 Often asymptomatic, in later stages visual field loss

Fundoscopy, retinal photography

 Medical: optimize glycaemic control

Laser photocoagulation: can prevent progression from proliferative retinopathy

HYPERTENSIVE RETINOPATHY

P In its simplest form, the classical account of hypertensive retinopathy (Keith–Wagener–Barker, see Box 6.2) describes 4 grades

Box 6.2 KEITH–WAGENER–BARKER CLASSIFICATION OF HYPERTENSIVE RETINOPATHY

- *Grade I*: arteriolar narrowing
- *Grade II*: arteriovenous nipping
- *Grade III*: flame-shaped haemorrhages
- *Grade IV*: optic disc swelling + macular oedema

(Rx) Blood pressure control

(Cx) Irreversible visual impairment or damage to the optic nerve or macula

CATARACT

(P) Opacification of the crystalline lens

(A) May be congenital (e.g. maternal rubella) or acquired (e.g. trauma)

Risk factors include ↑ age, diabetes mellitus, steroid therapy, trauma, chronic uveitis

(Sy) Blurred vision, haloes, glare

(Si) Loss of red reflex, brownness in the lens under slit lamp examination, a white pupil if the cataract is advanced

(Rx) Commonest operation in ophthalmology

Operation performed when vision affects activities of daily living for a given patient

Two main techniques are phacoemulsification (see Information box) and occasionally extracapsular extraction

---

INFORMATION BOX: PHACOEMULSIFICATION

In 'phaco', the cataract is divided into portions by an ultrasound cutter and the diseased lens removed. Then an intraocular lens implant is placed within the eye.
    A small incision is used so stitches are not routinely necessary. The operation is usually done under local anaesthetic and patients go home the same day.
    See Fig. 6.2

With extracapsular surgery a large corneal incision is made and the lens is removed in one piece

The wound is stitched and a lens implant placed into the eye

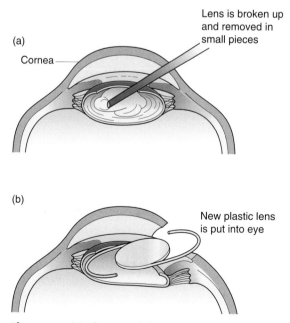

(a)

Cornea

Lens is broken up and removed in small pieces

(b)

New plastic lens is put into eye

Figure 6.2 (a) Phacoemulsification; (b) posterior chamber lens implantation (copyright © 2001 McKesson Health Solutions LLC. Used with permission of the University of Michigan Health System, April 2006)

NERVE PALSIES

Six muscles are found around the eye.

These are the lateral rectus (*ab*duction), medial rectus (*ad*duction), superior rectus (elevation), inferior rectus (depression), superior oblique (depression combined with adduction, intortion), and inferior oblique (elevation combined with adduction, extortion).

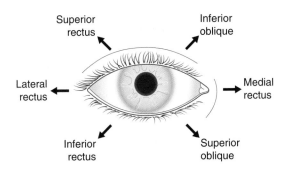

Figure 6.3 The muscles of eye movement (right eye illustrated)

All muscles are innervated by the III nerve, except the lateral rectus (VI nerve) and superior oblique (IV nerve): LR6 SO4 is the time-honoured mnemonic.

THIRD NERVE PALSY
 Cardiovascular risk factors (hypertension, diabetes, dyslipidaemia, smoking), ↑intracranial pressure, vasculitis, demyelination

Si The eye is ptotic and in a 'down and out' (depressed and abducted) position
This orientation follows from suppressed elevation (superior rectus and inferior oblique) and the unopposed pull of the lateral rectus (underactive medial rectus)
The upper lid is ptotic because the III nerve also drives the levator palpebrae superioris (elevates the eyelid)

FOURTH NERVE PALSY
A Head trauma, congenital IV palsy, cardiovascular risk factors
Si The affected eye is elevated relative to the fellow eye in primary position (the depressive effect of the superior oblique is missing)
The eye is unable to look 'down and in', a position which tests the primary direction of pull for the superior oblique

SIXTH NERVE PALSY
A Cardiovascular risk factors, ↑intracranial pressure (false localizing sign), demyelination, vasculitis
 The eye cannot abduct beyond the midline

THE OPTIC DISC

It is customary to describe the optic disc in terms of cup, colour and contour (the 3 Cs).

CUP

- The cup refers to the bowl-shaped depression in the centre of the disc.
- There is anatomical and pathological variation in the size of the cup.
- In advanced disc swelling the cup disappears because of the gross swelling of the neuroretinal rim.
- In advanced glaucoma the cup is enlarged because the neuroretinal rim is destroyed.

COLOUR

- The colour of the disc is usually a pink–red, with the cup being a whitish area in the centre.
- Many conditions can produce pallor of the optic disc.
- These include a space-occupying intracranial lesion, previous optic neuritis, B_{12}/folate deficiency, glaucoma, infarction of the optic disc.

CONTOUR

- The contour refers to the margin of the disc.
- The normal disc has pulsating vessels on the disc (the retinal veins, to which pressure waves in the eye are transmitted).
- Venous pulsation is abolished in the swollen disc (however note that in 20 per cent of the population there is no detectable physiological venous pulsation).
- The margin can be become indistinct in the early stages of disc swelling (especially nasally).
- With advanced disc swelling the margin of the disc can become blurred.
- With establishment of disc swelling it is seen that the plane of the optic disc is raised compared to the surrounding retina, an important sign that confirms swelling.

Box 6.3 CAUSES OF OPTIC DISC SWELLING

- *Local*:
    - optic neuritis
    - optic disc vasculitis (e.g. giant cell arteritis)
    - disc infarction
- *Systemic*:
    - intracranial space-occupying lesion
    - severe hypertension
    - leukaemic cell infiltration
    - metastases

OPTIC DISC ATROPHY

- **P** Loss of fibres within the optic nerve
- **A** *Local*: advanced glaucoma, intracranial space-occupying lesion (e.g. pituitary tumour), optic disc infarction (non-arteritic anterior ischaemic optic atrophy)
  Systemic: drugs, B_{12}/folate deficiency, tobacco, alcohol
- **Sy** Blurred vision, ↓ acuity, loss of colour vision

(Si) Pale optic disc
(Rx) Treatment of underlying cause if possible

OPTIC NEURITIS

(P) Inflammation of the optic nerve
(A) Common first presentation of multiple sclerosis, rarely infections
(Si) Loss of vision, eye pain, impairment of colour vision, swollen optic disc
(Ix) Magnetic resonance imaging (MRI)
(Rx) Treat underlying cause

Oncology

Kirstin Satherley

INTRODUCTION

- **P** Malignancy = ability of a tumour to demonstrate local invasion, lymph node involvement and distant (metastatic) spread, usually via blood or lymphatics
- **A** >250 000 new cases per annum of cancer in UK
  - 1 in 3 people will be diagnosed with cancer in their lifetime
  - 1 in 4 people will die from cancer
  - Prevalence ~2 per cent of population in UK (1.2 million people)
- **Px** Survival rates are improving with earlier diagnosis and better treatment

Table 7.1 Incidence of cancers in the UK

Cancer	% Incidence in UK (2000)
Male	
Prostate	20 (27 149)
Lung	17 (23 245)
Large bowel	14 (18 956)
Bladder	6 (7 876)
Stomach	5 (6 088)
Female	
Breast	30 (40 467)
Large bowel	12 (16 344)
Lung	11 (15 165)
Ovary	5 (6 734)
Endometrium	4 (6 002)

Adapted from Cancer Research UK. *Cancerstats Monograph 2004*. London: Cancer Research UK, 2004

Table 7.2 Deaths from all cancer types in the UK

Cancer type	% of all deaths (male and female, 2000)
Lung	22
Bowel	10
Breast	8
Prostate	6
Oesophagus	5

Adapted from Cancer Research UK. *Cancerstats Monograph 2004*. London: Cancer Research UK, 2004

AETIOLOGY AND MECHANISM OF DISEASE

- There is usually no single factor that leads to the development of a tumour in a particular patient – it is a combination of genetic risk factors and environmental influences
- *Environmental risk factors*: e.g. cigarette smoking (accounts for >30 per cent all cancers), UV light, alcohol, obesity, asbestos, hydrocarbons, aflatoxin, viruses (Epstein–Barr virus (EBV), hepatitis B virus (HBV), human papillomavirus (HPV), human T-cell lymphotropic virus type 1 (HTLV-1)
- *Genetic risk factors*: e.g. BRCA1 and 2 genes for breast cancer. 'Oncogenes' account for an increased risk of certain cancers in 1st degree relatives
- *Hereditary conditions* that predispose to the development of malignancy e.g. familial polyposis coli
- The combination of genetic/environmental factors leads to structural changes in the DNA molecule, which in turn leads to uncontrolled cell division and tumour growth

TREATMENT OPTIONS

- *Intention of treatment*:
  - curative
  - palliative (i.e. symptom control/prolong life but non-curative)
- *Modes of treatment*:
  - surgery
  - chemotherapy
  - radiotherapy (RT)
  - or a combination
- Factors affecting choice of treatment: tumour stage (often TNM – tumour, node metastases), performance status, co-morbidity, age, patient preference
- Patients should be discussed at a multidisciplinary team (MDT) meeting (physician, surgeon, oncologist, pathologist, radiologist as minimum)

PRINCIPLES OF SURGERY

CURATIVE

- Surgery is the mainstay for curative treatment: if at operation the tumour can be removed with margins that are clear of microscopic disease
- Can be combined with 'neoadjuvant' or 'adjuvant' chemotherapy or RT:
  - neoadjuvant treatment is given *before* surgery to reduce tumour bulk and limit disease to enable surgery to be curative, or allow less complex surgery to be performed
  - adjuvant treatment is given *after* surgery to decrease the chance of tumour recurrence
- The presence of metastases no longer precludes curative surgery: disease can be firstly downstaged with chemotherapy and then metastasectomy attempted e.g. limited liver resection

PALLIATIVE

- Surgery can also be a palliative measure, providing significant symptom relief and prolonging life expectancy without removing all the tumour e.g. to relieve duodenal obstruction from carcinoma of the head of the pancreas or resection of solitary brain metastasis

HISTOLOGY

- Surgery allows sufficient tissue to be obtained for histological diagnosis (further tissue analysis determines further treatment options e.g. oestrogen receptor status in breast cancer)
- Accurate staging e.g. Dukes' staging of bowel cancer, lymph node involvement
- Immediate histological examination intra-operatively can inform the surgeon if enough tissue has been resected

NON-SURGICAL INTERVENTION

CHEMOTHERAPY

PRINCIPLES OF CHEMOTHERAPY

- Chemotherapy targets and damages any rapidly dividing cells – hence destroying malignant cells preferentially
- Non-malignant cells that rapidly divide are also affected, which partly accounts for the toxic side-effects of chemotherapy (e.g. hair follicles, gastrointestinal [GI] tract mucosa, bone marrow)
- Normal cell cycle: allows increased number, growth, replacement and repair of cells
- Chromosomes contain DNA and have a regulatory role in cell division
- Chemotherapy affects cell cycle at different points
- Cell regulation is a complex process: if DNA damage is detected then cell cycle is halted and repair of cell damage or apoptosis (cell suicide) occurs
- Drug resistance commonly develops – if tumour recurs after initial treatment then an alternative regime will be needed

CLASSIFICATION OF CHEMOTHERAPY AGENTS

- *Modes of administration*: intravenous (i.v.) bolus, i.v. infusion, oral, intrathecal, intravesical
- *Single versus combination regimes*: combination often has superior effect
- *Side effects*: e.g. nausea and vomiting, change in bowel habit, immunosuppression, skin reactions, alopecia, neuropathy

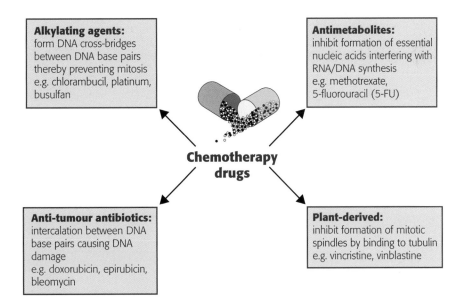

Alkylating agents:
form DNA cross-bridges between DNA base pairs thereby preventing mitosis e.g. chlorambucil, platinum, busulfan

Antimetabolites:
inhibit formation of essential nucleic acids interfering with RNA/DNA synthesis e.g. methotrexate, 5-fluorouracil (5-FU)

Chemotherapy drugs

Anti-tumour antibiotics:
intercalation between DNA base pairs causing DNA damage e.g. doxorubicin, epirubicin, bleomycin

Plant-derived:
inhibit formation of mitotic spindles by binding to tubulin e.g. vincristine, vinblastine

Figure 7.1 Chemotherapy drugs

RADIOTHERAPY

PRINCIPLES OF RADIOTHERAPY

- Radiation (X-rays or radioactivity) causes cell death or damage. RT directs radiation at the tumour, usually by means of an external beam carefully positioned outside the patient
- Occasionally a radioactive source is placed close to the tumour in the patient (brachytherapy)
- RT can be used for curative and palliative cases. Curative cases tend to receive a course of treatment over weeks; palliative cases receive either a single treatment or a short course
- RT causes irreversible DNA damage directly or indirectly by generating toxic free radicals. Process is oxygen dependent and the most important factor in cell killing – hence need to keep haemoglobin (Hb) >10 g/dL during course of RT treatment
- Effects of RT are dependent on dose, tumour size, tumour growth rate, hypoxia, anaemia and performance status of patient including co-morbidity
- Side-effects are divided into early (<90 days) and late (90+ days)

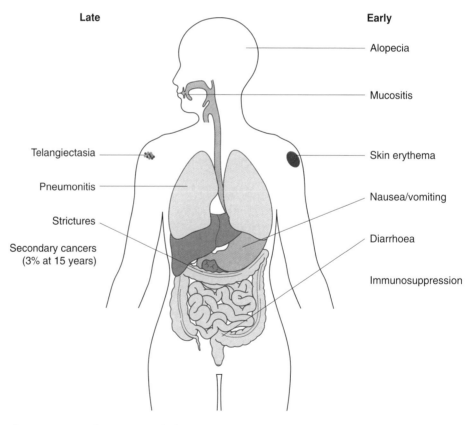

Figure 7.2 Complications of radiotherapy

OTHER TREATMENTS

- *Hormones*: e.g. tamoxifen (anti-oestrogen receptor in breast cancer), goserelin
- *Biological*: e.g. monoclonal antibodies – rituximab for non-Hodgkin's lymphoma – causes B cell lysis
- *Pharmacological*: e.g. bisphosphonates – decrease pathological fractures in bone metastases. They work in areas of high osteoclastic activity, reducing osteolysis and may allow healing of some osteolytic metastases

ONCOLOGICAL EMERGENCIES: DIAGNOSIS AND TREATMENT

NEUTROPENIC SEPSIS

P Occurs when neutrophil count $<1.0 \times 10^9/L$

Typically occurs 10–14 days after chemotherapy

A Common organisms: Gram +ve/–ve bacilli, fungal, atypical (e.g. *Pneumocystis carinii* pneumonia [PCP])

S Pyrexia >38°C, rigors, rash, inflammation, infective symptoms, hypotension

Ix Blood cultures (peripheral and central from *in situ* line)

Urine/sputum/stool/swab from i.v. line for microscopy, culture and sensitivity (MC&S)

Chest X-ray (CXR)

Rx Many patients with curative disease die as a result of delayed diagnosis of neutropenia – do not wait for full blood count (FBC) before giving antibiotics! Prompt detection and treatment are essential to prevent complications. Can be fatal

Start empirical broad-spectrum antibiotics early (according to hospital protocol)

Consider use of granulocyte cell-stimulating factors (G-CSF) to ↑ white cell count (WCC)

Close liaison with microbiologist essential

Barrier nursing

HYPERCALCAEMIA OF MALIGNANCY

P Calcium level often >3.5 mmol/L

Due to bone metastases or ectopic parathyroid hormone (PTH) secretion

Sy Malaise, nausea and vomiting, drowsiness, constipation

Si Polydipsia, polyuria, dehydration, fits, psychosis, confusion, coma

Rx *Hydration*: 3–4 L 0.9 per cent normal saline per 24 h

Bisphosphonates: pamidronate, zolendronic acid

Stop thiazide diuretics (cause hypercalcaemia), consider loop diuretics

Treat malignancy

Response expected within 3–5 days

SPINAL CORD COMPRESSION

P 70 per cent thoracic; 20 per cent lumbosacral; 10 per cent cervical

S Back pain, weakness, upper motor neurone and sensory signs (sensory level may be identifiable), urinary retention, faecal incontinence

Ix Plain X-rays of spine

Urgent magnetic resonance imaging (MRI) scan (definitive diagnosis)

Rx Consider suitability for neurosurgical decompression

Dexamethasone 4–8mg qds

RT to involved area on urgent basis

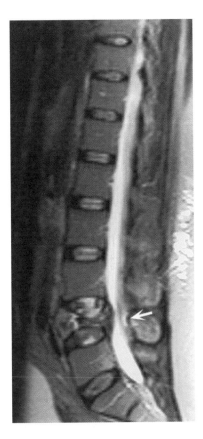

Figure 7.3 MRI (T$_2$W): vertebral deposit at L4 causing thecal compression

SUPERIOR VENA CAVA OBSTRUCTION

 80 per cent lung cancer; 17 per cent lymphoma

Distended thoracic/neck veins, dyspnoea, oedema, feeling of fullness in head, headache, ↑jugular venous pressure (JVP), plethoric face, tachypnoea

Sputum cytology

CXR

Computed tomography (CT) of the thorax

Dexamethasone 4 mg qds

Chemotherapy (small cell carcinoma and lymphoma)

RT (squamous cell carcinoma)

Superior vena cava stent insertion (palliative measure only)

SYMPTOM CONTROL

- Common symptoms include pain, nausea and vomiting, constipation, diarrhoea, symptomatic ascites ± pleural effusions, anxiety and depression

PAIN

 Multifaceted: physical, psychological, social

 Assess pain carefully and treat underlying cause

Regular analgesia instead of prn is more effective

Analgesics are more powerful when given prophylactically

Various routes: oral, intramuscular, i.v., subcutaneous (s.c.), *per rectum*, epidural, i.v./s.c. infusion

Methods of providing pain relief (see World Health Organization pain ladder, Fig. 7.4):

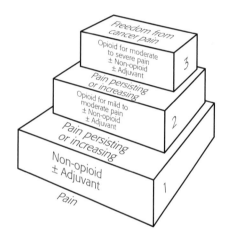

Figure 7.4 World Health Organization analgesic pain ladder:
- Step 1: non-opioid e.g. aspirin, paracetamol, non-steroidal anti-inflammatory drugs
- Step 2: weak opioid e.g. codeine, dihydrocodeine ± non-opioid
- Step 3: strong opioid e.g. morphine ± non-opioid
- Adjuvants: antidepressants, steroids, anti-epileptic drugs

(Reproduced with kind permission from WHO)

- starting dose of strong opioids is dependent on previous analgesia used and hepatic and renal function
- remember there is no upper limit in opiate dose when treating neoplastic pain

Bone pain can be reduced by RT, orthopaedic fixation of pathological fractures, bisphosphonates

Role of pain team – can advise if patient is intolerant to opioid of choice, drug interactions, adjuvant treatment

NAUSEA AND VOMITING

- Often treatment of the underlying cause is sufficient e.g. hypercalcaemia
- Anti-emetics include antihistamines e.g. cyclizine, hyoscine or dopamine antagonists e.g. haloperidol
- Gastric stasis is best treated with peripheral dopamine antagonists e.g. metoclopramide, domperidone
- Early chemotherapy-related nausea can be controlled with serotonin (5-HT$_3$) antagonists e.g. ondansetron

CONSTIPATION

- Prevention in high-risk patients is the key
- Regular use of laxatives e.g. bisacodyl, sodium docusate
- If patient is on regular opioids, then co-danthramer is the most effective and the dose is titrated against soft stools
- If the rectum is full start with glycerin suppositories and consider enemas

DIARRHOEA

- Mainstay of management is rehydration and loperamide
- If infection is the cause, antibiotics may be commenced
- RT-related diarrhoea responds to loperamide and codeine phosphate

CARE OF THE TERMINALLY ILL PATIENT

- The dying phase is an important stage in a patient's illness and is often the stage which most affects the family and carers
- A holistic approach is essential – physical, psychological, social and spiritual needs must be addressed
- Symptom control is a priority of palliative care. Many of the common symptoms are described above but they also include terminal agitation which is best treated with midazolam or haloperidol
- Medications are often administered to a terminally ill patient by means of a syringe driver which:
  - allows a continuous infusion of medication to be given subcutaneously over a 24 hour period
  - avoids the need for venous access and is suitable for the unconscious patient
  - often contains a 'cocktail' of medication such as diamorphine, metoclopramide, hyoscine and midazolam
- Multidisciplinary team approach is essential – early involvement of specialist nurses and doctors
- Consider continuing care in the hospice or at home with Macmillan support

CARDIOPULMONARY RESUSCITATION STATUS

- Often a difficult subject for the patient, family and medical team. If a patient shows signs of deterioration and further medical treatment is likely to be unsuccessful then early discussion with the patient can help establish their wishes regarding resuscitation
- Some patients with metastatic disease still have a good prognosis in that they will have a life expectancy of many years (e.g. hormone/chemotherapy-responsive breast cancer or prostate cancer), and these patients may wish to be considered for resuscitation
- If there is an identifiable cause e.g. septic shock secondary to neutropenic sepsis or cardiac arrhythmia secondary to chemotherapy, then resuscitation can be justified as these are often reversible conditions
- There is no right or wrong answer and each individual case is different
- Ultimately, the final decision regarding resuscitation status is made at consultant level, but this should obviously take into account the patient's wishes
- Any decision not to resuscitate should be clearly documented in the medical notes and conveyed to the nursing staff

Public health

Kinesh Patel

STATISTICS

BASIC DEFINITIONS

- *Prevalence*: the proportion of a population with a disease at any particular time e.g. 13 in 100 children suffer from asthma
- *Incidence*: the number of new cases of a disease in a particular time period e.g. 33 in 100 000 people are diagnosed with stomach cancer every year
- *Mortality*: the proportion of people who die from a disease e.g. 40 per cent of people who are diagnosed with meningococcal septicaemia die
- *Standardized mortality ratio*: the rate of deaths in one population compared with national averages corrected for age, sex, social class etc.
- *Relative risk*: the risk of developing disease for one population with an exposure compared with a population without the exposure e.g. smokers are 20 times more likely to contract lung cancer than non-smokers
- *Number needed to treat (NNT)*: the number of people receiving a treatment for one person to derive a benefit e.g. after myocardial infarction 18 people need to take an angiotensin-converting enzyme (ACE) inhibitor to prevent one heart attack (NNT = 18)

TESTING

- No diagnostic test is 100 per cent perfect
- To gauge the accuracy of a test there are several measures used to assess how reliable it is
- These are often expressed as mathematical formulae (see Table 8.1):

Table 8.1 Accuracy of tests

	Test positive	Test negative
Have disease	a (true positive)	b (false negative)
Do not have disease	c (false positive)	d (true negative)

- It is often easier to understand what each of the terms mean if the question they seek to answer is remembered (see Table 8.2)

Table 8.2 Definitions used in testing

Term	Question	Formula
Sensitivity	'If a group of people have a disease, what percentage of them will test positive?'	$\dfrac{a}{a+b}$
Specificity	'If a group of people do not have a disease, what percentage of them will test negative?'	$\dfrac{d}{c+d}$
Positive predictive value (PPV)	'If a person has a positive test result, what chance do they have of actually having the disease?'	$\dfrac{a}{a+c}$
Negative predictive value (NPV)	'If a person has a negative test result, what chance do they have of not having the disease?'	$\dfrac{d}{b+d}$

- Knowing the sensitivity and specificity of a test will influence the decision whether or not to perform it – a test with low sensitivity will not help confirm a diagnosis
- The best tests have sensitivities and specificities near 100 per cent
- The predictive values indicate the likelihood of a positive or negative screening test result meaning the presence or absence of the disease
- Knowing the predictive value will influence the view that an individual does or does not have the disease, once the test result is known

BIAS

- Bias is a systematic flaw with data collection, leading to results from the analysis of the data being incorrect
- Statistical analysis cannot be used to compensate for the effects of bias
- Whereas increasing the size of the study will decrease random error, this will not affect the level of bias
- The best way to avoid bias is effective study design e.g. double-blind placebo-controlled randomized trial
- There are several types of bias:
  - *selection bias:* those included in a trial do not reflect a typical population e.g. excluding those aged over 65 years from a study into ischaemic heart disease
  - *information bias:* wrongly assigning trial participants incorrect diagnoses/exposures

- *reporting bias:* cases with disease remember exposures better than those who are disease free
- *interviewer bias:* an interviewer may ask patients with disease more questions about exposures than those who are disease free
- *loss to follow-up:* if a significant proportion of trial participants drop out as time progresses, then the final data cannot be reliably interpreted
- *lead time bias:* earlier diagnosis of a condition results in an apparently longer survival time (see Fig. 8.1)
- *publication bias:* trials with positive results are much more likely to be published

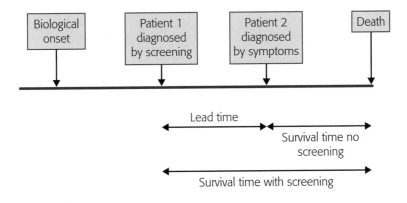

Figure 8.1 Lead time bias

SCREENING

The purpose of screening is to discover latent disease in apparently healthy individuals so that treatment can be offered to improve prognosis

---

Box 8.1 CRITERIA FOR SCREENING

- The condition screened for should be an important health problem
- The natural history of the disease should be well understood
- There should be a detectable pre-clinical stage with a long latent phase
- The pre-clinical stage must have a high prevalence in the target population
- There should be a test for the condition that is:
  - cheap
  - acceptable
  - reliable
  - easy to administer
- There should be a treatment for the disease at the preclinical stage that:
  - is effective
  - is sustainable
  - reduces morbidity and mortality

STUDIES

- There are many different ways of studying populations
- Generally prospective trials are more powerful than retrospective studies
- Randomization is a strategy to decrease the effect of bias on data
- Double-blinding (neither the doctor nor the patient know the treatment given) is another effective way to increase the validity of data
- The two major types of clinical study are case–control and cohort studies
- Case–control studies take a known case of the disease and then match one or more controls to that person to see what differences exist between the affected and unaffected groups
- Cohort studies take two separate groups and follow them

Table 8.3 Advantages and disadvantages of cohort and case–control studies

Type	Case–control study	Cohort study
Advantages	Quick/inexpensive	Valuable for rare exposures
	Easy to study diseases with long latent periods	Can reveal temporal relationship between exposure and disease
	Good for evaluation of rare diseases	Minimizes bias in exposure ascertainment
	Can examine multiple aetiological factors for a single disease	Allows direct incidence calculation
Disadvantages	Inefficient for evaluation of rare exposures	Inefficient for evaluation of rare diseases
	Cannot compute incidence rates in exposed and unexposed individuals	Prospective: expensive and time-consuming
	The temporal relationship between exposure and disease may be difficult to establish	Retrospective: availability of adequate records
	Problems with recall and selection bias	Losses to follow-up can affect results

EVIDENCE-BASED MEDICINE

- Modern medicine is now increasingly based on the principle that patient care should be based on evidence from high-quality trials
- There are difference qualities of evidence, in order of decreasing reliability:
  - meta-analysis (data from several high-quality trials analysed together)
  - multiple randomized control trials
  - single randomized control trial
  - non-randomized control trial
  - uncontrolled trial
  - retrospective studies (case–control, cross-sectional)
  - case series
  - case report
- For rarer conditions, generally there is less high-quality evidence available for clinical use

INFECTIOUS DISEASES

NOTIFIABLE DISEASES

- Some diseases have to be notified to the authorities when diagnosed so that outbreaks of disease can be contained and contacts traced
- It is the responsibility of the doctor to ensure that the local consultant in communicable disease control is notified of any of the diseases shown in Box 8.2

Box 8.2 NOTIFIABLE DISEASES

- Acute encephalitis
- Acute poliomyelitis
- Anthrax
- Cholera
- Diphtheria
- Dysentery
- Food poisoning
- Leptospirosis
- Malaria
- Measles
- Meningitis (meningococcal, pneumococcal, *Haemophilus influenzae*, viral, other)
- Meningococcal septicaemia (without meningitis)
- Mumps
- Ophthalmia neonatorum

- Paratyphoid fever
- Plague
- Rabies
- Relapsing fever
- Rubella
- Scarlet fever
- Smallpox
- Tetanus
- Tuberculosis
- Typhoid fever
- Typhus fever
- Viral haemorrhagic fever
- Viral hepatitis (hepatitis A, hepatitis B, hepatitis C, other)
- Whooping cough
- Yellow fever

Source: Health Protection Agency. Diseases notifiable (to Local Authority Proper Officers) under the Public Health (Infectious Diseases) Regulations 1988. www.phls.co.uk/infections/topics_az/noids/noidlist.htm

---

- The Public Health Laboratory Service aims to identify outbreaks of disease with these data and prevent further spread

VACCINATION

- Vaccination aims to protect individuals from disease by exposing them to an attenuated version of the pathogen

---

Box 8.3 DISEASES FOR WHICH VACCINES ARE CURRENTLY AVAILABLE

Anthrax	Pertussis
Diphtheria	Pneumococcus
Haemophilus influenzae type B	Rabies
Hepatitis A	Rubella
Hepatitis B	Smallpox
Influenza	TB (BCG)
Japanese B encephalitis	Tetanus
Measles	Tick-borne encephalitis
Meningococcus (A and C)	Typhoid
Mumps	Yellow fever

- High levels of population vaccination prevent the spread of disease by reducing the number of cases – so-called herd immunity
- For effective herd immunity, over 95 per cent of the population needs to be vaccinated
- Recent public concerns over the safety of vaccines has led to a general decrease in the level of herd immunity, with consequent increases in cases of diseases such as measles

Table 8.4 Routine childhood immunization schedule

	DTaP/Hib/ polio	Men C	MMR	dTaP/ polio	BCG	Td/polio
Birth					✓*	
2 months	✓	✓				
3 months	✓	✓				
4 months	✓	✓				
13 months			✓			
3–5 years			✓	✓		
13–18 years						✓

DTaP: diphtheria, tetanus, pertussis; Hib: *Haemophilus influenzae* type B; Men C: Meningococcus type C; MMR: mumps, measles, rubella; BCG: Bacille Calmette–Guérin (tuberculosis); *at-risk groups only

Index